2. Scrambled eggs with spinach and tomatoes

Ingredient:

• 3 large eggs
• 1 cup fresh spinach, chopped
• 1/2 cup cherry tomatoes, halved
• 1 tbsp olive oil
• 1 tbsp grated Parmesan cheese (optional)
• Salt and pepper to taste

Instructions:

1. In a small bowl, whisk the eggs until well combined.

2. Heat the olive oil in a non•stick skillet over medium heat.

3. Add the chopped spinach and sauté for 1•2 minutes until wilted.

4. Pour in the whisked eggs and let them sit for 30 seconds to set the bottom.

5. Use a spatula to gently push the eggs from the side of the pan towards the center, tilting the pan to allow the uncooked egg to flow to the edges.

6. Once the eggs are mostly set but still a bit moist, stir in the halved cherry tomatoes.

7. Continue cooking and stirring until the eggs are fully cooked but still soft.

8. Remove from heat and sprinkle with Parmesan cheese (if using).

9. Season with salt and pepper to taste.

Nutrition Information (per serving):
• Calories: 190
• Total Carbs: 5g
• Fiber: 2g
• Net Carbs: 3g
• Protein: 16g
• Fat: 13g

This scrambled egg dish is an excellent option for individuals over 50 with diabetes. The spinach and tomatoes provide fiber, vitamins, and antioxidants, while the eggs offer high•quality protein to help keep blood sugar stable.

3. Oatmeal with almond butter and flax seeds

Ingredient:

- 1/2 cup old·fashioned rolled oats
- 1 cup unsweetened almond milk
- 1 tbsp almond butter
- 1 tbsp ground flax seeds
- 1/2 tsp cinnamon
- 1 tsp honey (optional)

Instructions:

1. In a small saucepan, combine the rolled oats and almond milk.

2. Bring the mixture to a simmer over medium heat, stirring occasionally, until the oats are cooked and the mixture has thickened, about 5·7 minutes.

3. Remove the oatmeal from heat and stir in the almond butter, ground flax seeds, and cinnamon until well combined.

4. If desired, drizzle the oatmeal with a small amount of honey for a touch of sweetness.

Nutrition Information (per serving):
- Calories: 280
- Total Carbs: 28g
- Fiber: 7g
- Net Carbs: 21g
- Protein: 10g
- Fat: 15g

This oatmeal dish is an excellent choice for individuals over 50 with diabetes. The rolled oats provide complex carbs and fiber to help regulate blood sugar levels, while the almond butter and flax seeds add healthy fats and protein to promote satiety. The cinnamon may also help improve insulin sensitivity. The honey is optional, as the natural sweetness of the almond milk and oats can be enough for many people.

As we age, our bodies undergo a myriad of changes, many of which can significantly impact our health and well-being. One of the most common challenges faced by individuals over 50 is the increased risk of developing type 2 diabetes and prediabetes. Managing these conditions effectively is crucial to maintaining a healthy, active lifestyle and preventing further health complications. **"The Complete Diabetic Diet After 50"** is designed to be your comprehensive guide on this journey, offering over 110 delicious, low-sugar and low-carb recipes, along with a practical 60-day meal plan tailored specifically for those navigating life with prediabetes and type 2 diabetes.

This book is more than just a collection of recipes; it's a roadmap to healthier living. It starts with an in-depth exploration of diabetes, shedding light on its causes, symptoms, and the critical importance of diet in managing blood sugar levels. Understanding the role of carbohydrates and sugars in our diet is fundamental to controlling diabetes, and this guide provides clear, accessible explanations to help you make informed dietary choices.

Our carefully curated recipes are crafted to not only support your health goals but also to satisfy your taste buds. From hearty breakfasts to delectable dinners and everything in between, each recipe is designed with your nutritional needs in mind. We believe that eating well shouldn't mean sacrificing flavor, and our diverse range of dishes ensures that you'll never get bored with your meal plan.

In addition to recipes, this book features a structured 60-day meal plan, making it easy to adopt and maintain a balanced diet. This plan is flexible and can be tailored to fit your lifestyle, whether you're cooking for yourself or for a family. Each day is mapped out with specific meals and snacks, providing you with a stress-free approach to meal planning and preparation.

"The Complete Diabetic Diet After 50" is your trusted companion in the quest for better health. It's about empowering you with the knowledge and tools needed to take control of your diet and, by extension, your diabetes. By embracing the guidance and recipes within these pages, you are taking a significant step towards a healthier, more vibrant life. Let's embark on this journey together and transform the way you eat, one delicious meal at a time.

1. Greek yogurt with berries and chia seeds

Ingredient:

- 1 cup plain Greek yogurt (low•fat or non•fat)
- 1/2 cup mixed berries (such as blueberries, raspberries, and/or blackberries)
- 1 tbsp chia seeds

Instructions:

1. Spoon the Greek yogurt into a bowl.

2. Top the yogurt with the mixed berries.

3. Sprinkle the chia seeds over the top.

Nutrition Information (per serving):
- Calories: 180
- Total Carbs: 15g
- Fiber: 5g
- Net Carbs: 10g
- Protein: 18g
- Fat: 5g

This recipe is a great option for individuals over 50 with diabetes. The Greek yogurt provides protein and probiotics, the berries offer antioxidants and fiber, and the chia seeds add healthy omega•3 fatty acids. The carb content is moderate and the fiber helps to slow the absorption of sugars. Be sure to choose plain, unsweetened Greek yogurt to keep the sugar content low.

4. Avocado toast on whole grain bread

Ingredient:
- 2 slices of whole grain or sprouted bread
- 1/2 ripe avocado, mashed
- 1 tbsp lemon juice
- 1/4 tsp garlic powder
- Salt and pepper to taste
- Optional toppings: sliced tomatoes, crumbled feta, red pepper flakes

Instructions:
1. Toast the whole grain bread until lightly golden.

2. In a small bowl, mash the avocado with the lemon juice, garlic powder, salt, and pepper until well combined.

3. Spread the mashed avocado evenly over the toasted bread slices.

4. Top with any desired additional toppings, such as sliced tomatoes, crumbled feta, or a sprinkle of red pepper flakes.

Nutrition Information (per serving):
- Calories: 220
- Total Carbs: 22g
- Fiber: 7g
- Net Carbs: 15g
- Protein: 6g
- Fat: 13g

This avocado toast is an excellent option for individuals over 50 with diabetes. The whole grain bread provides complex carbs and fiber to help manage blood sugar levels, while the avocado offers healthy monounsaturated fats, fiber, and nutrients like potassium. The lemon juice and garlic add flavor without the need for added salt or sugar. This dish can be customized with additional toppings to suit individual preferences.

5. Cottage cheese with fresh peaches and walnuts

Ingredient:

- 1 cup low•fat or non•fat cottage cheese
- 1 medium fresh peach, sliced
- 2 tbsp chopped walnuts
- 1 tsp honey (optional)
- Cinnamon (to taste)

Instructions:

1. In a bowl, place the cottage cheese.

2. Top the cottage cheese with the sliced fresh peach.

3. Sprinkle the chopped walnuts over the peaches.

4. If desired, drizzle a small amount of honey over the top.

5. Lightly dust with cinnamon.

Nutrition Information (per serving):
- Calories: 220
- Total Carbs: 15g
- Fiber: 3g
- Net Carbs: 12g
- Protein: 20g
- Fat: 10g

This cottage cheese and peach dish is an excellent option for individuals over 50 with diabetes. The cottage cheese provides a good source of protein to help stabilize blood sugar levels, while the fresh peach offers natural sweetness and fiber. The walnuts add healthy fats and a satisfying crunch. The honey is optional, as the natural sweetness of the peach may be enough for many people. This dish can be enjoyed as a snack or light meal.

6. Smoothie with kale. cucumber. and green apple

Ingredient:

• 1 cup unsweetened almond milk
• 1 cup packed kale leaves, stems removed
• 1/2 cup diced cucumber
• 1/2 green apple, cored and chopped
• 1 tbsp ground flaxseed
• 1 tsp honey (optional)
• Ice cubes (as needed)

Instructions:

1. In a high•speed blender, combine the almond milk, kale, cucumber, green apple, and ground flaxseed.

2. Blend on high speed until the mixture is smooth and creamy.

3. If desired, add a small amount of honey to sweeten the smoothie.

4. Add ice cubes as needed to reach your desired consistency.

Nutrition Information (per serving):
• Calories: 150
• Total Carbs: 18g
• Fiber: 5g
• Net Carbs: 13g
• Protein: 5g
• Fat: 7g

This smoothie is an excellent choice for individuals over 50 with diabetes. The kale and cucumber provide a nutrient•dense base, while the green apple adds natural sweetness and fiber. The flaxseed contributes healthy omega•3 fatty acids. The almond milk keeps the carb count low and provides a creamy texture. The honey is optional, as the apple may provide enough sweetness for many people.

This smoothie is a great way to incorporate more vegetables and fruits into your diet in a diabetic•friendly way. It can be enjoyed as a snack or light meal.

7. Quinoa porridge with mixed berries

Ingredient:

- 1/2 cup uncooked quinoa, rinsed
- 1 1/2 cups unsweetened almond milk
- 1/4 tsp cinnamon
- 1/4 tsp vanilla extract
- 1/2 cup mixed berries (such as blueberries, raspberries, and blackberries)
- 1 tbsp chopped walnuts (optional)
- 1 tsp honey (optional)

Instructions:

1. In a small saucepan, combine the rinsed quinoa and almond milk. Bring the mixture to a boil over medium heat.

2. Once boiling, reduce the heat to low, cover, and simmer for 15•20 minutes, stirring occasionally, until the quinoa is cooked and the mixture has thickened.

3. Remove the quinoa porridge from heat and stir in the cinnamon and vanilla extract.

4. Transfer the quinoa porridge to a bowl and top with the mixed berries, chopped walnuts (if using), and a drizzle of honey (if desired).

Nutrition Information (per serving):
- Calories: 250
- Total Carbs: 35g
- Fiber: 7g
- Net Carbs: 28g
- Protein: 8g
- Fat: 9g

This quinoa porridge is an excellent choice for individuals over 50 with diabetes. Quinoa is a whole grain that is high in fiber and protein, which can help regulate blood sugar levels. The mixed berries provide antioxidants and additional fiber, while the cinnamon may help improve insulin sensitivity. The walnuts and honey are optional, but they can add healthy fats and a touch of sweetness if desired.

This porridge can be enjoyed for breakfast or as a healthy snack, and it's a great way to incorporate more whole grains and nutrient•dense foods into your diabetic•friendly diet.

8. Chia pudding with unsweetened almond milk and strawberries

Ingredient:

• 1/4 cup chia seeds
• 1 cup unsweetened almond milk
• 1 tsp vanilla extract
• 1/4 tsp cinnamon
• 1 cup fresh strawberries, sliced

Instructions:

1. In a medium bowl, whisk together the chia seeds, almond milk, vanilla extract, and cinnamon until well combined.

2. Cover the bowl and refrigerate for at least 2 hours, or overnight, stirring occasionally, until the chia seeds have thickened the mixture into a pudding•like consistency.

3. When ready to serve, top the chia pudding with the sliced fresh strawberries.

Nutrition Information (per serving):
• Calories: 200
• Total Carbs: 18g
• Fiber: 10g
• Net Carbs: 8g
• Protein: 6g
• Fat: 11g

This chia pudding is an excellent choice for individuals over 50 with diabetes. Chia seeds are high in fiber, protein, and healthy omega•3 fatty acids, which can help regulate blood sugar levels. The unsweetened almond milk keeps the carb count low, while the fresh strawberries provide natural sweetness and additional fiber.

The cinnamon in this recipe may also help improve insulin sensitivity. This chia pudding can be enjoyed as a healthy breakfast, snack, or dessert. It's a versatile and nutrient•dense option for a diabetic•friendly diet.

9. Whole grain toast with smoked salmon and avocado

Ingredient:

• 2 slices of whole grain or sprouted bread, toasted
• 2 oz smoked salmon
• 1/2 ripe avocado, sliced
• 1 tbsp lemon juice
• 1 tsp capers (optional)
• Salt and pepper to taste

Instructions:

1. Toast the whole grain bread until lightly golden.

2. Arrange the smoked salmon and avocado slices on top of the toasted bread.

3. Drizzle the lemon juice over the avocado.

4. If desired, sprinkle the capers over the top.

5. Season with salt and pepper to taste.

Nutrition Information (per serving):
• Calories: 300
• Total Carbs: 20g
• Fiber: 7g
• Net Carbs: 13g
• Protein: 18g
• Fat: 18g

This whole grain toast with smoked salmon and avocado is an excellent choice for individuals over 50 with diabetes. The whole grain bread provides complex carbs and fiber to help manage blood sugar levels, while the smoked salmon offers high•quality protein and healthy omega•3 fatty acids. The avocado adds heart•healthy monounsaturated fats and additional fiber.

The lemon juice and optional capers provide a flavorful contrast without the need for added salt or sugar. This dish can be enjoyed as a satisfying breakfast, lunch, or snack, and it's a great way to incorporate nutrient•dense foods into a diabetic•friendly diet.

10. Poached eggs on a bed of sautéed greens

Ingredient:
• 2 cups mixed greens (such as spinach, kale, and Swiss chard), chopped
• 1 tbsp olive oil
• 2 cloves garlic, minced
• 2 large eggs
• 1 tbsp white vinegar
• Salt and pepper to taste

Instructions:
1. In a large skillet, heat the olive oil over medium heat. Add the chopped greens and minced garlic. Sauté for 3•5 minutes, until the greens are wilted and tender.

2. Reduce the heat to low and create two small wells in the greens for the eggs.

3. Carefully crack the eggs into the wells.

4. In a small saucepan, bring 2•3 inches of water to a gentle simmer and add the white vinegar.

5. Carefully transfer the poached eggs from the saucepan to the bed of sautéed greens using a slotted spoon.

6. Season the dish with salt and pepper to taste.

Nutrition Information (per serving):
• Calories: 220
• Total Carbs: 8g
• Fiber: 3g
• Net Carbs: 5g
• Protein: 16g
• Fat: 15g

This poached egg and sautéed greens dish is an excellent choice for individuals over 50 with diabetes. The greens provide a nutrient•dense base, while the poached eggs offer high•quality protein to help stabilize blood sugar levels. The olive oil and garlic add flavor without the need for added salt or sugar.

This dish is a great way to incorporate more leafy greens into your diet, which are rich in vitamins, minerals, and antioxidants. It can be enjoyed for breakfast, lunch, or dinner as part of a balanced, diabetic•friendly meal plan.

11. Almond flour pancakes with fresh blueberries

Ingredient:

- 1 cup almond flour
- 2 large eggs
- 1/4 cup unsweetened almond milk
- 1 tsp baking powder
- 1/4 tsp cinnamon
- 1/4 tsp vanilla extract
- 1 cup fresh blueberries
- 1 tbsp butter or coconut oil for cooking

Instructions:

1. In a medium bowl, whisk together the almond flour, eggs, almond milk, baking powder, cinnamon, and vanilla extract until a smooth batter forms.

2. Gently fold in the fresh blueberries.

3. Heat a non•stick skillet or griddle over medium heat and melt the butter or coconut oil.

4. Scoop the batter onto the hot surface, forming pancakes about 3•4 inches in diameter.

5. Cook for 2•3 minutes per side, or until golden brown.

6. Serve the almond flour pancakes warm, with additional fresh blueberries if desired.

Nutrition Information (per serving, 2 pancakes):
- Calories: 280
- Total Carbs: 15g
- Fiber: 6g
- Net Carbs: 9g
- Protein: 12g
- Fat: 20g

These almond flour pancakes are an excellent choice for individuals over 50 with diabetes. Almond flour is low in carbs and high in healthy fats and protein, which can help regulate blood sugar levels. The fresh blueberries add natural sweetness, fiber, and antioxidants without significantly increasing the carb content.

This recipe is a great way to enjoy a satisfying and nutrient•dense breakfast or brunch option as part of a diabetic•friendly diet. The pancakes can be topped with a small amount of sugar•free syrup or a dollop of plain Greek yogurt if desired.

12. Tofu scramble with bell peppers and onions

Ingredient:

- 1 block (14 oz) firm or extra•firm tofu, crumbled
- 1 tbsp olive oil
- 1/2 cup diced bell peppers (any color)
- 1/2 cup diced onion
- 1 tsp ground turmeric
- 1/2 tsp garlic powder
- 1/4 tsp ground cumin
- Salt and pepper to taste
- 2 tbsp chopped fresh parsley (optional)

Instructions:

1. In a large non•stick skillet, heat the olive oil over medium heat.

2. Add the diced bell peppers and onions to the skillet. Sauté for 5•7 minutes, until the vegetables are tender.

3. Crumble the tofu into the skillet with the vegetables. Add the turmeric, garlic powder, cumin, salt, and pepper.

4. Stir the mixture well and continue cooking for 5•7 minutes, stirring occasionally, until the tofu is heated through and the flavors are combined.

5. Remove from heat and stir in the chopped parsley, if using. Serve the tofu scramble warm.

Nutrition Information (per serving):
- Calories: 180
- Total Carbs: 8g
- Fiber: 3g
- Net Carbs: 5g
- Protein: 16g
- Fat: 11g

This tofu scramble is an excellent choice for individuals over 50 with diabetes. Tofu is a great source of plant•based protein, and the bell peppers and onions provide fiber, vitamins, and antioxidants. The spices add flavor without the need for added salt or sugar.

This dish can be enjoyed for breakfast, lunch, or dinner, and it's a versatile option that can be customized with additional vegetables or herbs to suit your preferences. Serve it on its own or with a side of whole grain toast for a complete and balanced diabetic•friendly meal.

13. Buckwheat pancakes with sugar-free syrup

Ingredient:

- 1 cup buckwheat flour
- 1 tsp baking powder
- 1/4 tsp baking soda
- 1/4 tsp cinnamon
- 1 large egg
- 1 cup unsweetened almond milk
- 1 tbsp melted coconut oil or unsalted butter
- 1/2 tsp vanilla extract
- Sugar•free maple syrup (for serving)

Instructions:

1. In a medium bowl, whisk together the buckwheat flour, baking powder, baking soda, and cinnamon.

2. In a separate bowl, beat the egg. Then stir in the almond milk, melted coconut oil or butter, and vanilla extract.

3. Pour the wet ingredients into the dry ingredients and stir just until combined (do not overmix).

4. Heat a non•stick skillet or griddle over medium heat. Lightly grease the surface with a small amount of coconut oil or butter.

5. Scoop the batter onto the hot surface, forming pancakes about 3•4 inches in diameter.
6. Cook for 2•3 minutes per side, or until golden brown. Serve the buckwheat pancakes warm, drizzled with sugar•free maple syrup.

Nutrition Information (per serving, 2 pancakes):
- Calories: 220
- Total Carbs: 24g
- Fiber: 4g
- Net Carbs: 20g
- Protein: 8g
- Fat: 10g

These buckwheat pancakes are an excellent choice for individuals over 50 with diabetes. Buckwheat is a gluten•free, low•glycemic grain that is high in fiber and protein, which can help regulate blood sugar levels. The sugar•free maple syrup provides sweetness without the added sugars found in traditional syrups.

14. Breakfast burrito with eggs. black beans. and salsa

Ingredient:

• 2 large eggs, scrambled
• 1/2 cup canned black beans, rinsed and drained
• 2 tbsp mild salsa
• 1 whole wheat or low•carb tortilla
• 1 tbsp shredded cheddar cheese (optional)
• Salt and pepper to taste

Instructions:

1. In a small non•stick skillet, scramble the eggs over medium heat until cooked through. Season with a pinch of salt and pepper.

2. In a separate bowl, mix the rinsed and drained black beans with the salsa.

3. Lay the tortilla on a flat surface. Spoon the scrambled eggs down the center of the tortilla.

4. Top the eggs with the black bean and salsa mixture.

5. If desired, sprinkle the shredded cheddar cheese over the top.

6. Fold the bottom of the tortilla up, then fold in the sides and roll up tightly to create a burrito.

Nutrition Information (per serving):
• Calories: 300
• Total Carbs: 35g
• Fiber: 8g
• Net Carbs: 27g
• Protein: 18g
• Fat: 10g

This breakfast burrito is an excellent choice for individuals over 50 with diabetes. The whole wheat or low•carb tortilla provides complex carbs and fiber, while the eggs offer high•quality protein to help stabilize blood sugar levels. The black beans add additional fiber and plant•based protein, and the salsa provides flavor without added sugars.

The optional cheddar cheese adds a creamy texture and a boost of calcium. This burrito can be enjoyed for breakfast, brunch, or even a light lunch, and it's a great way to incorporate nutrient•dense ingredients into a diabetic•friendly meal.

15. Spinach and mushroom frittata

Ingredient:

- 8 large eggs
- 1/4 cup unsweetened almond milk
- 1 tbsp olive oil
- 8 oz sliced mushrooms
- 2 cups fresh spinach, chopped
- 2 tbsp grated Parmesan cheese
- 1/4 tsp garlic powder
- Salt and pepper to taste

Instructions:

1. Preheat your oven to 375°F.

2. In a medium bowl, whisk together the eggs and almond milk. Season with a pinch of salt and pepper. In a 9•inch oven•safe non•stick skillet, heat the olive oil over medium heat.

3. Add the sliced mushrooms and sauté for 3•4 minutes, until they start to soften. Add the chopped spinach and continue cooking for 2•3 minutes, until the spinach is wilted.

4. Pour the egg mixture over the mushrooms and spinach. Sprinkle the Parmesan cheese and garlic powder over the top.

5. Transfer the skillet to the preheated oven and bake for 18•22 minutes, or until the frittata is set and lightly golden on top. Remove the frittata from the oven and let it cool for a few minutes before slicing and serving.

Nutrition Information (per serving):
- Calories: 180
- Total Carbs: 5g
- Fiber: 2g
- Net Carbs: 3g
- Protein: 16g
- Fat: 12g

This spinach and mushroom frittata is an excellent choice for individuals over 50 with diabetes. The eggs provide high•quality protein, while the spinach and mushrooms offer fiber, vitamins, and antioxidants. The small amount of Parmesan cheese adds flavor without significantly increasing the carb or fat content.

16. Overnight oats with chia seeds and raspberries

Ingredient:

- 1/2 cup old•fashioned rolled oats
- 1 cup unsweetened almond milk
- 1 tbsp chia seeds
- 1/2 tsp vanilla extract
- 1/4 tsp cinnamon
- 1/2 cup fresh or frozen raspberries

Instructions:

1. In a medium•sized bowl or mason jar, combine the rolled oats, almond milk, chia seeds, vanilla extract, and cinnamon. Stir well to mix.

2. Cover the bowl or seal the mason jar and refrigerate overnight, or for at least 4 hours.

3. When ready to serve, stir the overnight oats and top with the fresh or frozen raspberries.

Nutrition Information (per serving):
- Calories: 250
- Total Carbs: 30g
- Fiber: 9g
- Net Carbs: 21g
- Protein: 8g
- Fat: 10g

This overnight oats recipe is an excellent choice for individuals over 50 with diabetes. The rolled oats provide complex carbs and fiber to help regulate blood sugar levels, while the chia seeds add healthy omega•3 fatty acids and additional fiber.

The raspberries offer natural sweetness, antioxidants, and more fiber. The cinnamon may also help improve insulin sensitivity. This dish is a convenient and nutrient•dense breakfast or snack option that can be prepared in advance.

You can adjust the amount of almond milk or add a small amount of honey or vanilla Greek yogurt if you prefer a creamier texture or slightly sweeter flavor. This recipe is a great way to incorporate more fiber•rich and nutrient•dense foods into a diabetic•friendly diet.

17. Pumpkin spice protein smoothie

Ingredient:

- 1/2 cup unsweetened almond milk
- 1/2 cup canned pumpkin puree
- 1 scoop vanilla protein powder (about 20•25g)
- 1 tbsp ground flaxseed
- 1/2 tsp pumpkin pie spice
- 1/4 tsp cinnamon
- 1 tsp vanilla extract
- Ice cubes (as needed)

Instructions:

1. In a high•speed blender, combine the almond milk, pumpkin puree, protein powder, ground flaxseed, pumpkin pie spice, cinnamon, and vanilla extract.

2. Blend on high speed until the mixture is smooth and creamy.

3. Add ice cubes as needed to reach your desired consistency.

Nutrition Information (per serving):
- Calories: 220
- Total Carbs: 16g
- Fiber: 5g
- Net Carbs: 11g
- Protein: 22g
- Fat: 8g

This pumpkin spice protein smoothie is an excellent choice for individuals over 50 with diabetes. The pumpkin puree provides fiber, vitamins, and antioxidants, while the protein powder helps to stabilize blood sugar levels and promote satiety.

The flaxseed adds healthy omega•3 fatty acids, and the pumpkin pie spice and cinnamon provide flavor without the need for added sugars. This smoothie can be enjoyed as a nutritious breakfast, snack, or post•workout recovery drink.

You can adjust the amount of protein powder or almond milk to suit your individual preferences and dietary needs. This recipe is a great way to incorporate more nutrient•dense, diabetic•friendly ingredients into your diet.

18. Veggie omelette with feta cheese

Ingredient:

- 3 large eggs
- 2 tbsp unsweetened almond milk
- 1/4 cup diced bell peppers
- 1/4 cup diced onions
- 1/2 cup spinach, chopped
- 2 tbsp crumbled feta cheese
- 1 tsp olive oil
- Salt and pepper to taste

Instructions:

1. In a small bowl, whisk together the eggs and almond milk. Season with a pinch of salt and pepper.

2. In a non•stick skillet, heat the olive oil over medium heat.

3. Add the diced bell peppers and onions to the skillet. Sauté for 2•3 minutes, until the vegetables start to soften.

4. Add the chopped spinach to the skillet and continue cooking for 1•2 minutes, until the spinach is wilted.

5. Pour the egg mixture into the skillet, tilting the pan to allow the eggs to evenly distribute.

6. As the eggs start to set, use a spatula to gently lift the edges, allowing the uncooked egg to flow underneath. When the eggs are mostly set but still slightly moist on top, sprinkle the crumbled feta cheese over the omelette. Fold the omelette in half and slide it onto a plate.

Nutrition Information (per serving):

- Calories: 220
- Total Carbs: 7g
- Fiber: 2g
- Net Carbs: 5g
- Protein: 18g
- Fat: 14g

This veggie omelette with feta cheese is an excellent choice for individuals over 50 with diabetes. The eggs provide high•quality protein to help stabilize blood sugar levels, while the bell peppers, onions, and spinach offer fiber, vitamins, and antioxidants.

19. Whole grain English muffin with peanut butter

Ingredient:

• 1 whole grain English muffin
• 2 tbsp natural peanut butter (no added sugar)
• 1 tsp chia seeds (optional)

Instructions:

1. Toast the whole grain English muffin until lightly golden.

2. Spread the natural peanut butter evenly over the toasted muffin.

3. If desired, sprinkle the chia seeds over the peanut butter.

Nutrition Information (per serving):
• Calories: 250
• Total Carbs: 25g
• Fiber: 6g
• Net Carbs: 19g
• Protein: 12g
• Fat: 13g

This whole grain English muffin with peanut butter is an excellent choice for individuals over 50 with diabetes. The whole grain muffin provides complex carbs and fiber to help regulate blood sugar levels, while the peanut butter offers a source of healthy fats and protein to promote satiety.

The optional chia seeds add additional fiber, protein, and omega•3 fatty acids, further enhancing the nutritional profile of this snack or light meal.

This recipe is a simple and satisfying option that can be enjoyed for breakfast or as a snack. It's a great way to incorporate whole grains, healthy fats, and protein into a diabetic•friendly diet.

Remember to choose a natural peanut butter without added sugars or oils to keep the carb and fat content in check.

20. Smoothie bowl with unsweetened coconut. kiwi. and chia seeds

Ingredient:

• 1 cup unsweetened almond milk
• 1 cup frozen mixed berries
• 1 kiwi, peeled and sliced
• 2 tbsp unsweetened shredded coconut
• 1 tbsp chia seeds
• 1 tsp vanilla extract
• 1/4 tsp cinnamon

Instructions:

1. In a high•speed blender, combine the almond milk, frozen mixed berries, vanilla extract, and cinnamon. Blend until smooth and creamy.

2. Pour the smoothie into a bowl.

3. Top the smoothie with the sliced kiwi, unsweetened shredded coconut, and chia seeds.

Nutrition Information (per serving):
• Calories: 250
• Total Carbs: 25g
• Fiber: 10g
• Net Carbs: 15g
• Protein: 6g
• Fat: 14g

This smoothie bowl is an excellent choice for individuals over 50 with diabetes. The frozen mixed berries provide natural sweetness, fiber, and antioxidants, while the kiwi adds more fiber and vitamin C.

The unsweetened coconut and chia seeds contribute healthy fats and additional fiber to help regulate blood sugar levels and promote feelings of fullness. The almond milk keeps the carb content low and provides a creamy base for the smoothie.

This recipe is a nutrient•dense and visually appealing option that can be enjoyed for breakfast or as a snack. It's a great way to incorporate more fiber•rich and antioxidant•rich foods into a diabetic•friendly diet.

21. Greek yogurt parfait with unsweetened granola

Ingredient:

- 1 cup plain Greek yogurt
- 1/2 cup fresh berries (such as blueberries, raspberries, or blackberries)
- 1/4 cup unsweetened granola
- 1 tsp honey (optional)

Instructions:

1. In a parfait glass or bowl, layer half of the Greek yogurt.

2. Top the yogurt with half of the fresh berries.

3. Sprinkle half of the unsweetened granola over the berries.

4. Repeat the layers, ending with the granola on top.

5. If desired, drizzle a small amount of honey over the top of the parfait.

Nutrition Information (per serving):
- Calories: 200
- Total Carbs: 18g
- Fiber: 4g
- Net Carbs: 14g
- Protein: 18g
- Fat: 6g

This Greek yogurt parfait with unsweetened granola is an excellent choice for individuals over 50 with diabetes. The Greek yogurt provides a good source of protein to help stabilize blood sugar levels, while the fresh berries offer fiber, vitamins, and antioxidants.

The unsweetened granola adds a crunchy texture and a boost of complex carbs and fiber without the added sugars found in many commercial granola products. The optional honey can provide a touch of sweetness, but the parfait is delicious without it.

This parfait is a versatile and nutrient•dense option that can be enjoyed for breakfast, as a snack, or even as a light dessert. It's a great way to incorporate more protein, fiber, and antioxidants into a diabetic•friendly diet.

22. Apple slices with almond butter

Ingredient:
- 1 medium apple, cored and sliced
- 2 tbsp natural almond butter (no added sugar)

Instructions:
1. Wash and slice the apple into thin wedges or slices.

2. Spread a small amount of almond butter (about 1•2 tsp) onto each apple slice.

Nutrition Information (per serving, 2•3 apple slices with 1 tbsp almond butter):
- Calories: 150
- Total Carbs: 12g
- Fiber: 3g
- Net Carbs: 9g
- Protein: 5g
- Fat: 10g

This simple snack of apple slices with almond butter is an excellent choice for individuals over 50 with diabetes. The apple provides natural sweetness, fiber, and antioxidants, while the almond butter offers healthy fats and protein to help regulate blood sugar levels.

The combination of the crisp apple and the creamy almond butter creates a satisfying and nutrient•dense snack. The fiber from the apple helps to slow the absorption of the natural sugars, and the protein and healthy fats from the almond butter can help promote feelings of fullness.

This snack is easy to prepare and can be enjoyed as a quick pick•me•up or as part of a larger diabetic•friendly meal. It's a great way to incorporate more fresh fruit and healthy fats into your diet.

Remember to choose a natural almond butter without added sugars or oils to keep the carb and fat content in check.

23. Steel•cut oats with cinnamon and chopped nuts

Ingredient:

- 1/2 cup steel•cut oats
- 1 1/2 cups unsweetened almond milk
- 1/4 tsp cinnamon
- 1 tbsp chopped walnuts or pecans
- 1 tsp honey (optional)

Instructions:

1. In a small saucepan, combine the steel•cut oats and almond milk.

2. Bring the mixture to a boil over medium heat, then reduce the heat to low and simmer, stirring occasionally, for 20•25 minutes, until the oats are tender and the mixture has thickened.

3. Remove the oats from heat and stir in the cinnamon.

4. Transfer the oatmeal to a bowl and top with the chopped nuts. If desired, drizzle a small amount of honey over the top.

Nutrition Information (per serving):
- Calories: 250
- Total Carbs: 30g
- Fiber: 6g
- Net Carbs: 24g
- Protein: 8g
- Fat: 12g

This steel•cut oats dish is an excellent choice for individuals over 50 with diabetes. Steel•cut oats are a whole grain that is higher in fiber and lower on the glycemic index compared to rolled oats, which can help regulate blood sugar levels.

The cinnamon may also help improve insulin sensitivity, and the chopped nuts provide healthy fats and additional fiber to promote feelings of fullness. The optional honey can add a touch of sweetness, but the dish is delicious without it.

This recipe is a comforting and nutrient•dense breakfast option that can be enjoyed on its own or with a side of fresh fruit. It's a great way to incorporate more whole grains, fiber, and healthy fats into a diabetic•friendly diet.

24. Millet porridge with dried apricots and almonds

Ingredient:

- 1/2 cup uncooked millet
- 2 cups unsweetened almond milk
- 1/4 tsp cinnamon
- 1/4 tsp vanilla extract
- 3 dried apricots, chopped
- 2 tbsp sliced almonds

Instructions:

1. In a medium saucepan, combine the millet and almond milk. Bring the mixture to a boil over medium heat.

2. Once boiling, reduce the heat to low, cover, and simmer for 20•25 minutes, stirring occasionally, until the millet is tender and the porridge has thickened.

3. Remove the porridge from heat and stir in the cinnamon and vanilla extract. Transfer the millet porridge to a bowl and top with the chopped dried apricots and sliced almonds.

Nutrition Information (per serving):
- Calories: 250
- Total Carbs: 30g
- Fiber: 5g
- Net Carbs: 25g
- Protein: 7g
- Fat: 10g

This millet porridge is an excellent choice for individuals over 50 with diabetes. Millet is a gluten•free whole grain that is high in fiber and protein, which can help regulate blood sugar levels.

The dried apricots provide natural sweetness and additional fiber, while the almonds add healthy fats and crunch. The cinnamon may also help improve insulin sensitivity.

This porridge is a warm and comforting breakfast option that can be enjoyed on its own or with a side of fresh fruit. It's a great way to incorporate more whole grains, fiber, and nutrient•dense ingredients into a diabetic•friendly diet.

You can adjust the amount of almond milk or add a small amount of honey if you prefer a creamier or slightly sweeter porridge.

25. Cottage cheese with cucumber and dill

Ingredient:

• 1 cup low•fat or non•fat cottage cheese
• 1/2 cup diced cucumber
• 1 tbsp chopped fresh dill
• 1 tsp lemon juice
• Salt and pepper to taste

Instructions:

1. In a small bowl, combine the cottage cheese, diced cucumber, chopped dill, and lemon juice.

2. Stir the ingredients together until well mixed. Season with a pinch of salt and pepper to taste.

Nutrition Information (per serving):
• Calories: 150
• Total Carbs: 8g
• Fiber: 1g
• Net Carbs: 7g
• Protein: 20g
• Fat: 3g

This cottage cheese with cucumber and dill is an excellent choice for individuals over 50 with diabetes. Cottage cheese is a great source of protein, which can help stabilize blood sugar levels. The cucumber provides fiber, vitamins, and hydration, while the fresh dill adds flavor without the need for added salt or sugar.

The lemon juice provides a refreshing tang and a small amount of vitamin C. This dish is a simple, yet nutrient•dense snack or light meal that can be enjoyed on its own or with a side of whole grain crackers or sliced bell peppers.

The combination of protein, fiber, and low•carb ingredients makes this recipe a great option for managing diabetes. It's a versatile and easy•to•prepare dish that can be customized with additional herbs or spices to suit your taste preferences.

26. Grilled chicken salad with mixed greens and balsamic vinaigrette

Ingredient:

- 2 tbsp balsamic vinegar
- 1 tbsp olive oil
- 1 tsp Dijon mustard
- 1 tsp honey (optional)
- Salt and pepper to taste
- 4 oz grilled chicken breast, sliced
- 2 cups mixed greens (such as spinach, kale, and arugula)
- 1/2 cup cherry tomatoes, halved
- 1/4 cup sliced cucumber
- 2 tbsp crumbled feta cheese

Instructions:

1. In a large salad bowl, combine the mixed greens, cherry tomatoes, and sliced cucumber.

2. Top the salad with the grilled chicken slices and crumbled feta cheese.

3. In a small bowl, whisk together the balsamic vinegar, olive oil, Dijon mustard, and honey (if using). Season with a pinch of salt and pepper. Drizzle the balsamic vinaigrette over the salad and toss gently to coat.

Nutrition Information (per serving):
- Calories: 300
- Total Carbs: 12g
- Fiber: 3g
- Net Carbs: 9g
- Protein: 32g
- Fat: 15g

This grilled chicken salad is an excellent choice for individuals over 50 with diabetes. The mixed greens provide a nutrient•dense base, while the grilled chicken offers high•quality protein to help regulate blood sugar levels.

The cherry tomatoes, cucumber, and balsamic vinaigrette add flavor, fiber, and antioxidants without significantly increasing the carb content. The optional honey in the dressing can provide a touch of sweetness, but the salad is delicious without it.

This salad is a great way to incorporate more lean protein, vegetables, and healthy fats into a diabetic•friendly diet. It can be enjoyed as a main dish or a side salad, and it's a versatile option that can be customized with additional toppings or dressings to suit your preferences.

27. Quinoa and black bean salad with lime dressing

Ingredient:

- 1 cup cooked quinoa, cooled
- 1 (15 oz) can black beans, rinsed and drained
- 1 cup diced bell peppers (any color)
- 1/2 cup diced red onion
- 1/4 cup chopped cilantro
- 2 tbsp lime juice
- 1 tbsp olive oil
- 1 tsp Dijon mustard
- 1/4 tsp cumin
- Salt and pepper to taste

Instructions:

1. In a large bowl, combine the cooked quinoa, black beans, diced bell peppers, red onion, and chopped cilantro.

2. In a small bowl, whisk together the lime juice, olive oil, Dijon mustard, and cumin. Season with a pinch of salt and pepper.

3. Pour the lime dressing over the quinoa and black bean mixture and toss gently to coat. Serve the salad chilled or at room temperature.

Nutrition Information (per serving):
- Calories: 220
- Total Carbs: 30g
- Fiber: 8g
- Net Carbs: 22g
- Protein: 9g
- Fat: 7g

This quinoa and black bean salad is an excellent choice for individuals over 50 with diabetes. Quinoa is a whole grain that is high in fiber and protein, which can help regulate blood sugar levels. The black beans provide additional fiber and plant·based protein.

The diced bell peppers, red onion, and cilantro add flavor, vitamins, and antioxidants, while the lime dressing provides a refreshing, tangy contrast without the need for added sugars.

28. Lentil soup with spinach and tomatoes

Ingredient:
- 1 cup dry brown or green lentils, rinsed
- 4 cups low•sodium vegetable or chicken broth
- 1 tbsp olive oil
- 1 onion, diced
- 3 cloves garlic, minced
- 2 cups diced tomatoes (canned or fresh)
- 2 cups fresh spinach, chopped
- 1 tsp dried thyme
- 1/2 tsp ground cumin
- Salt and pepper to taste

Instructions:
1. In a large pot, bring the broth to a boil over high heat. Add the rinsed lentils, reduce heat to medium•low, and simmer for 20•25 minutes, until the lentils are tender.

2. In a separate skillet, heat the olive oil over medium heat. Add the diced onion and sauté for 3•4 minutes, until translucent.

3. Add the minced garlic to the onions and cook for 1 minute, until fragrant.

4. Transfer the sautéed onions and garlic to the pot with the cooked lentils.

5. Stir in the diced tomatoes, chopped spinach, dried thyme, and ground cumin. Season with salt and pepper to taste.

6. Simmer the soup for an additional 5•10 minutes, until the spinach is wilted and the flavors have combined.

This lentil soup is an excellent choice for individuals over 50 with diabetes. Lentils are a great source of fiber and plant•based protein, which can help regulate blood sugar levels. The spinach and tomatoes provide additional fiber, vitamins, and antioxidants.

The combination of the hearty lentils, nutrient•dense vegetables, and flavorful spices makes this soup a satisfying and diabetic•friendly meal. It can be enjoyed on its own or with a side of whole grain bread or a small salad.

This recipe is easy to prepare and can be made in advance, making it a convenient option for busy weeknights or meal prepping. Adjust the seasoning to your taste preferences, and consider adding other vegetables or herbs to customize the soup to your liking.

29. Turkey and avocado wrap in a whole grain tortilla

Ingredient:

- 1 whole grain tortilla or wrap
- 3 oz sliced turkey breast
- 1/2 avocado, sliced
- 1 tbsp hummus
- 1/4 cup shredded lettuce
- 1 tbsp diced tomatoes
- Salt and pepper to taste

Instructions:

1. Lay the whole grain tortilla or wrap on a flat surface.

2. Spread the hummus evenly over the center of the tortilla.

3. Layer the sliced turkey breast, avocado slices, shredded lettuce, and diced tomatoes on top of the hummus.

4. Season with a pinch of salt and pepper.

5. Fold the bottom of the tortilla up, then fold in the sides and roll up tightly to create a wrap.

This turkey and avocado wrap is an excellent choice for individuals over 50 with diabetes. The whole grain tortilla provides complex carbs and fiber to help regulate blood sugar levels, while the turkey offers lean protein.

The avocado adds healthy monounsaturated fats, which can help promote feelings of fullness and support heart health. The hummus provides additional protein and fiber, and the lettuce and tomatoes contribute vitamins, minerals, and antioxidants.

This wrap is a well•balanced and portable option that can be enjoyed for lunch or as a snack. It's a great way to incorporate a variety of nutrient•dense ingredients into a diabetic•friendly meal.

You can customize the wrap by adding other vegetables, using a different type of protein, or adjusting the amount of hummus or avocado to suit your preferences.

30. Greek salad with grilled shrimp

Ingredient:
- 1 lb large shrimp, peeled and deveined
- 1 tbsp olive oil
- 1 tsp dried oregano
- 1/4 tsp salt
- 1/4 tsp black pepper
- 6 cups chopped romaine lettuce
- 1 cup cherry tomatoes, halved
- 1/2 cup sliced cucumber
- 1/4 cup crumbled feta cheese
- 2 tbsp sliced kalamata olives
- 2 tbsp red wine vinegar
- 1 tbsp lemon juice
- 1 tbsp extra·virgin olive oil
- 1 tsp Dijon mustard
- 1 garlic clove, minced

Instructions:
1. Preheat grill or grill pan to medium·high heat.

2. In a small bowl, toss the shrimp with 1 tbsp olive oil, oregano, salt, and pepper.

3. Grill the shrimp for 2·3 minutes per side, until opaque and cooked through. Set aside.

4. In a large salad bowl, combine the romaine lettuce, cherry tomatoes, cucumber, feta cheese, and olives.

5. In a small bowl, whisk together the red wine vinegar, lemon juice, 1 tbsp olive oil, Dijon mustard, and garlic.

6. Drizzle the dressing over the salad and toss to coat. Top the salad with the grilled shrimp and serve.

This recipe is diabetic·friendly as it is low in carbs, high in protein and healthy fats from the shrimp and olive oil. The portion size is also appropriate for individuals over 50. Enjoy!

31. Zucchini noodles with pesto and cherry tomatoes

Ingredient:

- 3 medium zucchini, spiralized or julienned into noodles
- 1 cup cherry tomatoes, halved
- 1/4 cup basil pesto (store•bought or homemade)
- 2 tbsp grated Parmesan cheese
- 1 tbsp toasted pine nuts
- 1 tbsp fresh basil leaves, chopped
- 1/4 tsp salt
- 1/8 tsp black pepper

Instructions:

1. In a large bowl, combine the zucchini noodles, cherry tomatoes, pesto, Parmesan cheese, pine nuts, and chopped basil. Toss to coat evenly.

2. Season with salt and pepper and toss again.

3. Serve immediately.

This recipe is diabetic•friendly for a few reasons:

• Zucchini noodles are low in carbs and high in fiber, making them a great alternative to traditional pasta.

• Pesto is made with healthy fats from olive oil and pine nuts, which can help control blood sugar levels.

• Cherry tomatoes are a low•glycemic fruit that provides vitamins, minerals, and antioxidants.

• The portion size is appropriate for individuals over 50, as it is a light, veggie•based dish.

This dish is also easy to prepare and can be a quick, healthy meal for those with diabetes. Enjoy!

32. Tuna salad with mixed greens and olive oil dressing

Ingredient:
- 2 (5 oz) cans of tuna, drained and flaked
- 2 tbsp olive oil
- 1 tbsp lemon juice
- 1 tsp Dijon mustard
- 1/4 tsp salt
- 1/8 tsp black pepper
- 4 cups mixed greens
 (such as spinach, arugula, and kale)
- 1/2 cup cherry tomatoes, halved
- 2 tbsp sliced cucumber
- 1 tbsp crumbled feta cheese

Dressing:
- 2 tbsp extra•virgin olive oil
- 1 tbsp red wine vinegar
- 1 tsp Dijon mustard
- 1 tsp lemon juice
- 1/4 tsp dried oregano
- 1/8 tsp salt
- 1/8 tsp black pepper

Instructions:

1. In a small bowl, mix together the tuna, 2 tbsp olive oil, 1 tbsp lemon juice, 1 tsp Dijon mustard, salt, and pepper. Set aside.

2. In a large salad bowl, combine the mixed greens, cherry tomatoes, and sliced cucumber.

3. In a small bowl, whisk together all the dressing ingredients.

4. Add the tuna salad and feta cheese to the salad bowl. Drizzle the dressing over the top and toss gently to coat. Serve immediately.

This recipe is diabetic•friendly for the following reasons:

- Tuna is a lean protein that is low in carbs and high in healthy fats, which can help regulate blood sugar levels.
- The mixed greens provide fiber, vitamins, and minerals without adding many carbs.
- The olive oil•based dressing is a healthy fat that can also help control blood sugar.
- The portion size is appropriate for individuals over 50, as it is a light, nutrient•dense meal

33. Chickpea and vegetable stir•fry

Ingredient:

- 1 tbsp olive oil
- 1 cup diced onion
- 1 cup sliced mushrooms
- 1 cup diced bell pepper
- 1 cup diced zucchini
- 1 (15 oz) can chickpeas, rinsed and drained
- 2 cloves garlic, minced
- 1 tsp ground cumin
- 1/2 tsp paprika
- 1/4 tsp salt
- 1/8 tsp black pepper
- 2 cups baby spinach leaves
- 2 tbsp chopped fresh parsley

Sauce:
- 2 tbsp low•sodium soy sauce
- 1 tbsp rice vinegar
- 1 tsp honey
- 1 tsp sesame oil

Instructions:

1. In a large skillet or wok, heat the olive oil over medium•high heat.

2. Add the onion, mushrooms, bell pepper, and zucchini. Stir•fry for 5•7 minutes, until the vegetables are tender•crisp.

3. Add the chickpeas, garlic, cumin, paprika, salt, and pepper. Stir•fry for 2•3 minutes.

4. In a small bowl, whisk together the soy sauce, rice vinegar, honey, and sesame oil.

5. Add the spinach and parsley to the stir•fry. Pour the sauce over the top and toss to coat everything evenly.

6. Cook for 1•2 minutes, until the spinach is wilted and the sauce has thickened slightly. Serve immediately.

This recipe is diabetic•friendly for the following reasons:

• Chickpeas are a good source of fiber and protein, which can help regulate blood sugar levels.

• The vegetables provide a variety of vitamins, minerals, and antioxidants without adding many carbs.

• The sauce is made with low•sodium soy sauce, rice vinegar, and a small amount of honey, which keeps the carb and sodium content low.

• The portion size is appropriate for individuals over 50, as it is a balanced, nutrient•dense meal.

34. Cauliflower rice with grilled vegetables

Ingredient:
• 1 head of cauliflower, riced (about 4 cups)
• 1 zucchini, sliced into 1/2•inch thick rounds
• 1 yellow squash, sliced into 1/2•inch thick rounds
• 1 red bell pepper, sliced into 1•inch pieces
• 1 onion, sliced into 1/2•inch thick rounds
• 2 tbsp olive oil, divided
• 1 tsp dried oregano
• 1/2 tsp garlic powder
• 1/4 tsp salt
• 1/8 tsp black pepper
• 2 tbsp chopped fresh parsley

Dressing:
• 2 tbsp olive oil
• 1 tbsp red wine vinegar
• 1 tsp Dijon mustard
• 1 tsp lemon juice
• 1/4 tsp salt
• 1/8 tsp black pepper

Instructions:

1. Preheat grill or grill pan to medium•high heat.

2. In a large bowl, toss the zucchini, yellow squash, bell pepper, and onion with 1 tbsp of olive oil, oregano, garlic powder, salt, and pepper.

3. Grill the vegetables for 3•5 minutes per side, until tender and slightly charred. Remove from grill and set aside.

4. In a food processor, pulse the cauliflower florets until they resemble rice•sized grains.

5. In a large skillet, heat the remaining 1 tbsp of olive oil over medium heat. Add the cauliflower rice and cook for 5•7 minutes, stirring occasionally, until tender.

6. In a small bowl, whisk together the dressing ingredients.

7. Add the grilled vegetables and parsley to the cauliflower rice. Drizzle the dressing over the top and toss to coat. Serve immediately.

35. Spinach and strawberry salad with walnuts

Ingredient:

- 5 cups baby spinach leaves
- 1 cup sliced fresh strawberries
- 1/4 cup chopped walnuts
- 2 tbsp crumbled feta cheese
- 2 tbsp balsamic vinegar
- 1 tbsp extra•virgin olive oil
- 1 tsp Dijon mustard
- 1 tsp honey
- 1/4 tsp salt
- 1/8 tsp black pepper

Instructions:

1. In a large salad bowl, combine the baby spinach, sliced strawberries, chopped walnuts, and crumbled feta cheese.

2. In a small bowl, whisk together the balsamic vinegar, olive oil, Dijon mustard, honey, salt, and black pepper to make the dressing.

3. Drizzle the dressing over the salad and toss gently to coat. Serve immediately.

This salad is diabetic•friendly for the following reasons:

- Spinach is a nutrient•dense, low•carb green that provides fiber, vitamins, and minerals.

- Strawberries are a low•glycemic fruit that are high in antioxidants and fiber.

- Walnuts are a good source of healthy fats, protein, and fiber, which can help regulate blood sugar levels.

- The dressing is made with a small amount of honey and balsamic vinegar, which are lower in carbs compared to other sweeteners.

- The portion size is appropriate for individuals over 50, as it is a light, nutrient•dense meal.

This salad is easy to prepare and can be a refreshing, healthy option for those with diabetes. Enjoy!

36. Broccoli and cheddar soup

Ingredient:

- 2 tbsp unsalted butter
- 1 onion, diced
- 2 cloves garlic, minced
- 4 cups low•sodium chicken or vegetable broth
- 4 cups chopped broccoli florets
- 1 cup unsweetened almond milk
- 1 cup shredded low•fat cheddar cheese
- 1/4 tsp salt
- 1/8 tsp black pepper

Instructions:

1. In a large pot or Dutch oven, melt the butter over medium heat.

2. Add the diced onion and minced garlic. Cook for 3•5 minutes, until the onion is translucent.

3. Pour in the broth and add the chopped broccoli florets. Bring the mixture to a boil, then reduce heat and simmer for 10•15 minutes, until the broccoli Is tender.

4. Using an immersion blender or regular blender, puree the soup until smooth.

5. Return the pureed soup to the pot and stir in the unsweetened almond milk and shredded cheddar cheese. Cook for 2•3 minutes, until the cheese is melted and the soup is heated through.

6. Season with salt and black pepper. Serve hot.

This broccoli and cheddar soup is diabetic•friendly for the following reasons:

- Broccoli is a low•carb, high•fiber vegetable that provides essential vitamins and minerals.
- The use of low•fat cheddar cheese and unsweetened almond milk helps keep the fat and carb content in check.
- The portion size is appropriate for individuals over 50, as it is a nutrient•dense, filling soup.
- The soup is made without any added sugars or high•carb ingredients, making it a suitable option for those with diabetes.

37. Grilled salmon with a side of steamed asparagus

Ingredient:

- 4 (4 oz) salmon fillets
- 1 tbsp olive oil
- 1 tsp lemon zest
- 1 tbsp lemon juice
- 1 tsp Dijon mustard
- 1/4 tsp salt
- 1/8 tsp black pepper
- 1 lb asparagus, trimmed
- 1 tbsp unsalted butter

Instructions:

1. Preheat grill or grill pan to medium•high heat.

2. In a small bowl, whisk together the olive oil, lemon zest, lemon juice, Dijon mustard, salt, and pepper.

3. Place the salmon fillets on a plate and brush the top and sides with the lemon•mustard mixture.

4. Grill the salmon for 4•6 minutes per side, or until it flakes easily with a fork.

5. While the salmon is grilling, bring a medium saucepan of water to a boil. Add the asparagus and steam for 5•7 minutes, until tender•crisp.

6. Drain the asparagus and toss with the butter.

7. Serve the grilled salmon fillets with the steamed asparagus on the side.

This meal is diabetic•friendly for the following reasons:

- Salmon is a lean protein that is high in healthy omega•3 fatty acids, which can help regulate blood sugar levels.
- Asparagus is a low•carb, high•fiber vegetable that provides essential vitamins and minerals.
- The portion sizes are appropriate for individuals over 50, with the salmon fillet being around 4 oz and the asparagus being a generous side.
- The recipe uses minimal added fats and no added sugars, keeping the carb and calorie content in check.

38. Chicken and vegetable skewers

Ingredient:
- 1 lb boneless, skinless chicken breasts, cut into 1·inch cubes
- 1 red bell pepper, cut into 1·inch pieces
- 1 zucchini, cut into 1/2·inch thick rounds
- 1 red onion, cut into 1·inch pieces
- 2 tbsp olive oil
- 1 tbsp lemon juice
- 1 tsp dried oregano
- 1/2 tsp garlic powder
- 1/4 tsp salt
- 1/8 tsp black pepper

Instructions:
1. Preheat grill or grill pan to medium·high heat.

2. In a large bowl, combine the chicken cubes, bell pepper pieces, zucchini rounds, and onion pieces.

3. In a small bowl, whisk together the olive oil, lemon juice, oregano, garlic powder, salt, and black pepper.

4. Pour the marinade over the chicken and vegetables and toss to coat evenly.

5. Thread the chicken and vegetables onto skewers, alternating the ingredients.

6. Grill the skewers for 12·15 minutes, turning occasionally, until the chicken is cooked through and the vegetables are tender. Serve immediately.

This chicken and vegetable skewer recipe is diabetic·friendly for the following reasons:
- Chicken is a lean protein that is low in carbs and high in nutrients.

- The vegetables (bell pepper, zucchini, and onion) are low in carbs and high in fiber, vitamins, and minerals.

- The marinade is made with healthy fats (olive oil) and seasonings, without any added sugars.

- The portion size is appropriate for individuals over 50, as the skewers provide a balanced, nutrient·dense meal.

39. Stuffed bell peppers with ground turkey and quinoa

Ingredient:

- 1 tsp dried oregano
- 1/2 tsp ground cumin
- 1/4 tsp salt
- 1/8 tsp black pepper
- 1 cup low•sodium tomato sauce
- 1/2 cup shredded
low•fat mozzarella cheese

- 4 medium bell peppers, halved lengthwise and seeds removed
- 1 lb ground turkey
- 1 cup cooked quinoa
- 1 small onion, diced
- 2 cloves garlic, minced

Instructions:

1. Preheat oven to 375°F.

2. In a large skillet, cook the ground turkey over medium heat until browned and crumbled, about 5•7 minutes. Drain any excess fat.

3. Add the diced onion and minced garlic to the skillet. Cook for 2•3 minutes, until the onion is translucent.

4. Stir in the cooked quinoa, oregano, cumin, salt, and pepper. Mix well.

5. Arrange the bell pepper halves in a baking dish. Spoon the turkey•quinoa mixture evenly into the pepper halves.

6. Pour the tomato sauce over the stuffed peppers, making sure to coat the tops.

7. Cover the dish with foil and bake for 25•30 minutes, until the peppers are tender.

8. Remove the foil, sprinkle the mozzarella cheese over the tops of the peppers, and bake for an additional 5•10 minutes, until the cheese is melted and bubbly. Serve hot.

This stuffed bell pepper dish is diabetic•friendly for the following reasons:

- Ground turkey is a lean protein that is low in carbs and high in nutrients.
- Quinoa is a high•fiber, high•protein grain that can help regulate blood sugar levels.
- Bell peppers are a low•carb, nutrient•dense vegetable that provides fiber, vitamins, and minerals.
- The portion size is appropriate for individuals over 50, as the stuffed pepper halves make for a balanced, satisfying meal.
- The recipe uses minimal added fats and no added sugars, keeping the carb and calorie content in check.

40. Eggplant parmesan with a side salad

Ingredient:

Eggplant Parmesan:
• 1 medium eggplant,
sliced into 1/2•inch thick rounds
• 1 cup whole wheat breadcrumbs
• 1/2 cup grated Parmesan cheese
• 1 tsp dried oregano
• 1/2 tsp garlic powder
• 1/4 tsp salt
• 1/8 tsp black pepper
• 1 egg, beaten
• 1 cup low•sodium marinara sauce
• 1/2 cup shredded part•skim mozzarella cheese

Side Salad:
• 4 cups mixed greens (such as
spinach, arugula, and romaine)
• 1 cup cherry tomatoes, halved
• 1/4 cup sliced cucumber
• 1 tbsp olive oil
• 1 tbsp balsamic vinegar
• 1/4 tsp dried oregano
• 1/8 tsp salt
• 1/8 tsp black pepper

Instructions:

Eggplant Parmesan:
1. Preheat oven to 375°F. Line a baking sheet with parchment paper.

2. In a shallow bowl, combine the breadcrumbs, Parmesan, oregano, garlic powder, salt, and pepper.

3. Dip the eggplant slices in the beaten egg, then coat them in the breadcrumb mixture, pressing gently to adhere.

4. Arrange the breaded eggplant slices on the prepared baking sheet.

5. Bake for 20•25 minutes, flipping halfway, until the eggplant is tender and the breading is golden brown.

6. Spread the marinara sauce over the eggplant slices and sprinkle with the mozzarella cheese. Bake for an additional 5•10 minutes, until the cheese is melted and bubbly.

Side Salad:
1. In a large salad bowl, combine the mixed greens, cherry tomatoes, and sliced cucumber.

2. In a small bowl, whisk together the olive oil, balsamic vinegar, oregano, salt, and pepper. Drizzle the dressing over the salad and toss to coat.

41. Cobb salad with turkey bacon and blue cheese

Ingredient:

- 6 cups mixed greens (such as romaine, spinach, and arugula)
- 3 oz cooked turkey bacon, crumbled
- 1 hard·boiled egg, chopped
- 1/2 cup diced tomatoes
- 1/4 cup diced avocado
- 2 tbsp crumbled blue cheese
- 2 tbsp red wine vinegar
- 1 tbsp olive oil
- 1 tsp Dijon mustard
- 1/4 tsp salt
- 1/8 tsp black pepper

Instructions:

1. In a large salad bowl, combine the mixed greens, crumbled turkey bacon, chopped hard·boiled egg, diced tomatoes, and diced avocado.

2. In a small bowl, whisk together the red wine vinegar, olive oil, Dijon mustard, salt, and black pepper to make the dressing.

3. Drizzle the dressing over the salad and toss gently to coat.

4. Sprinkle the crumbled blue cheese over the top of the salad. Serve immediately.

This Cobb salad is diabetic·friendly for the following reasons:

- Mixed greens are low in carbs and high in fiber, vitamins, and minerals.

- Turkey bacon is a lean protein that is lower in fat and calories compared to regular bacon.

- Avocado provides healthy fats that can help regulate blood sugar levels.

- Blue cheese adds flavor without significantly increasing the carb or calorie content.

- The portion size is appropriate for individuals over 50, as it is a nutrient·dense, filling meal.

The dressing is made with a small amount of olive oil and Dijon mustard, which helps keep the carb and calorie content low. This Cobb salad is a great option for a healthy, satisfying meal for those with diabetes.

42. Spaghetti squash with marinara sauce and turkey meatballs

Ingredient:

Spaghetti Squash:
• 1 medium spaghetti squash, halved lengthwise and seeds removed

Turkey Meatballs:
• 1 lb ground turkey
• 1/4 cup whole wheat breadcrumbs
• 2 tbsp grated Parmesan cheese
• 1 egg, beaten
• 2 cloves garlic, minced
• 1 tsp dried oregano
• 1/4 tsp salt
• 1/8 tsp black pepper

Marinara Sauce:
• 1 (15 oz) can no•salt•added diced tomatoes
• 2 cloves garlic, minced
• 1 tsp dried oregano
• 1/4 tsp salt
• 1/8 tsp black pepper

Instructions:
1. Preheat oven to 400°F.

2. Place the spaghetti squash halves cut•side down on a baking sheet. Bake for 40•50 minutes, until tender when pierced with a fork.

3. While the squash is baking, prepare the turkey meatballs. In a medium bowl, combine the ground turkey, breadcrumbs, Parmesan, egg, garlic, oregano, salt, and pepper. Mix well and form into 12 equal•sized meatballs.

4. Place the meatballs on a separate baking sheet and bake for 20•25 minutes, until cooked through.

5. In a medium saucepan, combine the diced tomatoes, garlic, oregano, salt, and pepper. Bring to a simmer and cook for 5•7 minutes, stirring occasionally.

6. Use a fork to shred the spaghetti squash flesh into strands. Serve the spaghetti squash noodles topped with the marinara sauce and turkey meatballs

43. Thai chicken lettuce wraps

Ingredient:

- 1 lb ground chicken
- 2 tbsp low•sodium soy sauce
- 1 tbsp rice vinegar
- 1 tbsp lime juice
- 1 tsp honey
- 1 tsp sesame oil
- 1 tsp grated ginger
- 1/2 tsp red pepper flakes (optional)
- 2 cloves garlic, minced
- 1/4 cup chopped fresh cilantro
- 1/4 cup chopped green onions
- 12 large lettuce leaves (such as romaine or bibb)
- 1/4 cup chopped peanuts (optional)

Instructions:

1. In a large skillet or wok, cook the ground chicken over medium•high heat, breaking it up with a wooden spoon, until no longer pink, about 5•7 minutes.

2. In a small bowl, whisk together the soy sauce, rice vinegar, lime juice, honey, sesame oil, grated ginger, and red pepper flakes (if using).

3. Add the minced garlic to the cooked chicken and cook for 1 minute, until fragrant.

4. Pour the sauce mixture into the skillet with the chicken and stir to coat. Cook for 2•3 minutes, until the sauce has thickened slightly.

5. Remove the skillet from heat and stir in the chopped cilantro and green onions. To serve, spoon the chicken mixture into the lettuce leaves. Top with chopped peanuts, if desired.

This Thai chicken lettuce wrap recipe is diabetic•friendly for the following reasons:

- Ground chicken is a lean protein that is low in carbs and high in nutrients.
- The sauce is made with low•sodium soy sauce, rice vinegar, lime juice, and a small amount of honey, keeping the carb and sodium content in check.
- Lettuce leaves are a low•carb, high•fiber alternative to traditional wraps or tortillas.
- The portion size is appropriate for individuals over 50, as the lettuce wraps make for a light, yet satisfying meal.
- The optional peanuts provide a crunchy texture and healthy fats without significantly increasing the carb content.

44. Vegetable and tofu stir•fry with brown rice

Ingredient:

- 1 cup uncooked brown rice
- 1 block (14 oz) extra•firm tofu, diced
- 2 tbsp low•sodium soy sauce
- 1 tbsp rice vinegar
- 1 tsp sesame oil
- 1 tbsp olive oil
- 1 cup sliced mushrooms
- 1 cup broccoli florets
- 1 red bell pepper, sliced
- 1 cup snow peas
- 2 cloves garlic, minced
- 1 tsp grated fresh ginger
- 1/4 tsp red pepper flakes (optional)
- 2 tbsp chopped fresh cilantr

Instructions:

1. Cook the brown rice according to package instructions.

2. In a small bowl, combine the soy sauce, rice vinegar, and sesame oil. Set aside.

3. In a large skillet or wok, heat the olive oil over medium•high heat.

4. Add the diced tofu and cook for 3•4 minutes, until lightly browned on all sides. Transfer the tofu to a plate.

5. Add the mushrooms, broccoli, bell pepper, and snow peas to the skillet. Stir•fry for 5•7 minutes, until the vegetables are tender•crisp.

6. Add the garlic and ginger to the skillet and cook for 1 minute, until fragrant.

7. Return the tofu to the skillet and pour in the soy sauce mixture. Toss everything together and cook for 2•3 minutes, until the sauce has thickened slightly.

8. Remove from heat and stir in the chopped cilantro. Serve the vegetable and tofu stir•fry over the cooked brown rice.

This recipe is diabetic•friendly for the following reasons:

- Brown rice is a whole grain that is higher in fiber and nutrients compared to white rice.
- Tofu is a lean, plant•based protein that is low in carbs.
- The vegetables provide a variety of vitamins, minerals, and antioxidants without adding many carbs.
- The sauce is made with low•sodium soy sauce and a small amount of rice vinegar, keeping the sodium and carb content in check.
- The portion size is appropriate for individuals with diabetes, as the stir•fry and brown rice make for a balanced, nutrient•dense meal.

45. Kale and quinoa salad with cranberries and almonds

Ingredient:

- 1 cup cooked quinoa
- 4 cups chopped kale
- 1/2 cup dried cranberries
- 1/4 cup sliced almonds
- 2 tbsp olive oil
- 1 tbsp lemon juice
- 1 tsp Dijon mustard
- 1 tsp honey
- 1/4 tsp salt
- 1/8 tsp black pepper

Instructions:

1. In a large salad bowl, combine the cooked quinoa, chopped kale, dried cranberries, and sliced almonds.

2. In a small bowl, whisk together the olive oil, lemon juice, Dijon mustard, honey, salt, and black pepper to make the dressing.

3. Pour the dressing over the salad and toss to coat the ingredients evenly.

4. Let the salad sit for 5•10 minutes to allow the kale to soften and the flavors to meld. Serve immediately.

This kale and quinoa salad is diabetic•friendly for the following reasons:

• Kale is a nutrient•dense, low•carb green that provides fiber, vitamins, and minerals.

• Quinoa is a high•fiber, high•protein grain that can help regulate blood sugar levels.

• Dried cranberries are a low•glycemic fruit that adds sweetness without too many carbs.

• Almonds provide healthy fats and a crunchy texture without significantly increasing the carb content.

• The dressing is made with a small amount of olive oil, lemon juice, Dijon mustard, and a touch of honey, keeping the carb and calorie content in check.

• The portion size is appropriate for individuals over 50, as it is a nutrient•dense, filling salad.

46. Minestrone soup with kidney beans and vegetables

Ingredient:

- 1 tbsp olive oil
- 1 onion, diced
- 2 carrots, peeled and diced
- 2 celery stalks, diced
- 3 cloves garlic, minced
- 1 tsp dried oregano
- 1/4 tsp salt
- 1/8 tsp black pepper
- 1/2 tsp dried basil
- 1/4 tsp red pepper flakes (optional)
- 4 cups low•sodium vegetable or chicken broth
- 1 (15 oz) can no•salt•added diced tomatoes
- 1 (15 oz) can no•salt•added kidney beans, rinsed and drained
- 2 cups chopped kale or spinach
- 1/2 cup uncooked whole wheat elbow macaroni

Instructions:

1. In a large pot or Dutch oven, heat the olive oil over medium heat.

2. Add the diced onion, carrots, and celery. Cook for 5•7 minutes, stirring occasionally, until the vegetables are softened.

3. Stir in the minced garlic, dried oregano, dried basil, and red pepper flakes (if using). Cook for 1 minute, until fragrant.

4. Pour in the vegetable or chicken broth and the diced tomatoes. Bring the mixture to a boil.

5. Reduce the heat to medium•low and stir in the rinsed and drained kidney beans, chopped kale or spinach, and uncooked whole wheat elbow macaroni.

6. Simmer the soup for 15•20 minutes, until the pasta is tender. Season with salt and black pepper.Serve hot.

This minestrone soup is diabetic•friendly for the following reasons:

- Kidney beans are a good source of fiber and protein, which can help regulate blood sugar levels.
- The vegetables (onion, carrots, celery, kale/spinach) provide a variety of vitamins, minerals, and antioxidants without adding many carbs.
- Whole wheat pasta is a higher•fiber, lower•glycemic alternative to regular pasta.
- The recipe uses low•sodium broth and canned goods, keeping the sodium content in check.
- The portion size is appropriate for individuals over 50, as the soup makes for a nutrient•dense, filling meal.

47. Shrimp and avocado salad with citrus dressing

Ingredient:

- 1 lb cooked shrimp, peeled and deveined
- 1 avocado, diced
- 1 cup cherry tomatoes, halved
- 1/2 cup thinly sliced cucumber
- 2 tbsp chopped fresh cilantro
- 2 tbsp olive oil
- 2 tbsp fresh orange juice
- 1 tbsp fresh lime juice
- 1 tsp Dijon mustard
- 1/4 tsp salt
- 1/8 tsp black pepper

Instructions:

1. In a large salad bowl, combine the cooked shrimp, diced avocado, cherry tomatoes, sliced cucumber, and chopped cilantro.

2. In a small bowl, whisk together the olive oil, orange juice, lime juice, Dijon mustard, salt, and black pepper to make the dressing.

3. Drizzle the dressing over the salad and toss gently to coat. Serve immediately.

This shrimp and avocado salad is diabetic•friendly for the following reasons:

• Shrimp is a lean protein that is low in carbs and high in nutrients.

• Avocado provides healthy fats that can help regulate blood sugar levels.

• The vegetables (tomatoes, cucumber) are low in carbs and high in fiber, vitamins, and minerals.

• The citrus•based dressing is made with a small amount of olive oil, orange juice, and lime juice, keeping the carb and calorie content low.

• The portion size is appropriate for individuals over 50, as the salad makes for a light, yet satisfying meal.

48. Grilled chicken Caesar salad with a light dressing

Ingredient:

- 4 boneless, skinless chicken breasts
- 1 tbsp olive oil
- 1 tsp dried oregano
- 1/4 tsp salt
- 1 tsp Worcestershire sauce
- 1 clove garlic, minced
- 1/4 tsp salt
- 1/8 tsp black pepper

- 1/8 tsp black pepper
- 6 cups chopped romaine lettuce
- 2 tbsp grated Parmesan cheese
- 2 tbsp whole wheat croutons
- 2 tbsp plain Greek yogurt
- 1 tbsp lemon juice
- 1 tsp Dijon mustard

Instructions:

1. Preheat grill or grill pan to medium•high heat.

2. Brush the chicken breasts with olive oil and season with oregano, salt, and pepper.

3. Grill the chicken for 5•7 minutes per side, until cooked through. Allow to cool slightly, then slice or chop the chicken.

4. In a large salad bowl, combine the chopped romaine lettuce, grilled chicken, Parmesan cheese, and whole wheat croutons.

5. In a small bowl, whisk together the Greek yogurt, lemon juice, Dijon mustard, Worcestershire sauce, garlic, salt, and pepper to make the dressing. Drizzle the dressing over the salad and toss gently to coat. Serve immediately.

This grilled chicken Caesar salad is diabetic•friendly for the following reasons:

- Grilled chicken is a lean protein that is low in carbs and high in nutrients.

- Romaine lettuce is a low•carb, high•fiber green that provides essential vitamins and minerals.

- The dressing is made with Greek yogurt, lemon juice, and a small amount of Dijon mustard and Worcestershire sauce, keeping the carb and calorie content low.

- The portion of whole wheat croutons is small, providing a crunchy texture without significantly increasing the carb intake.

- The overall portion size is appropriate for individuals with diabetes, as it is a balanced, nutrient•dense meal.

49. Mediterranean chickpea salad with feta cheese

Ingredient:

• 1 (15 oz) can no•salt•added chickpeas, rinsed and drained
• 1 cup cherry tomatoes, halved
• 1/2 cup diced cucumber
• 1/4 cup diced red onion
• 1/4 cup crumbled feta cheese
• 2 tbsp chopped fresh parsley
• 2 tbsp olive oil
• 1 tbsp red wine vinegar
• 1 tsp Dijon mustard
• 1 tsp lemon juice
• 1/4 tsp dried oregano
• 1/8 tsp salt
• 1/8 tsp black pepper

Instructions:

1. In a large bowl, combine the rinsed and drained chickpeas, halved cherry tomatoes, diced cucumber, diced red onion, crumbled feta cheese, and chopped fresh parsley.

2. In a small bowl, whisk together the olive oil, red wine vinegar, Dijon mustard, lemon juice, dried oregano, salt, and black pepper to make the dressing.

3. Pour the dressing over the chickpea salad and toss gently to coat. Cover and refrigerate for at least 30 minutes to allow the flavors to meld. Serve chilled or at room temperature.

This Mediterranean chickpea salad is diabetic•friendly for the following reasons:
• Chickpeas are a good source of fiber and protein, which can help regulate blood sugar levels.

• The vegetables (tomatoes, cucumber, onion) provide a variety of vitamins, minerals, and antioxidants without adding many carbs.

• Feta cheese adds flavor without significantly increasing the fat or carb content.

• The dressing is made with a small amount of olive oil, vinegar, and lemon juice, keeping the carb and calorie content low.

• The portion size is appropriate for individuals with diabetes, as the salad makes for a light, yet satisfying meal

50. Roasted beet and goat cheese salad

Ingredient:

• 3 medium beets, peeled
and cut into 1•inch cubes
• 1 tbsp olive oil
• 1/4 tsp salt
• 1/8 tsp black pepper
• 1 tsp honey
• 1/4 tsp salt
• 1/8 tsp black pepper

• 5 cups mixed greens (such as
spinach, arugula, and kale)
• 2 oz crumbled goat cheese
• 2 tbsp chopped walnuts
• 2 tbsp balsamic vinegar
• 1 tbsp olive oil
• 1 tsp Dijon mustard

Instructions:

1. Preheat oven to 400°F.

2. Toss the cubed beets with 1 tbsp of olive oil, 1/4 tsp of salt, and 1/8 tsp of black pepper. Spread the beets on a baking sheet and roast for 25•30 minutes, until tender.

3. Allow the roasted beets to cool slightly.

4. In a large salad bowl, combine the mixed greens, roasted beets, crumbled goat cheese, and chopped walnuts.

5. In a small bowl, whisk together the balsamic vinegar, 1 tbsp of olive oil, Dijon mustard, honey, 1/4 tsp of salt, and 1/8 tsp of black pepper to make the dressing. Drizzle the dressing over the salad and toss gently to coat. Serve immediately.

This roasted beet and goat cheese salad is diabetic•friendly for the following reasons:

• Beets are a low•carb, high•fiber vegetable that provides essential vitamins and minerals. Goat cheese is a flavorful, lower•fat alternative to other cheeses.

• Walnuts provide healthy fats and a crunchy texture without significantly increasing the carb content.

• The dressing is made with a small amount of olive oil, balsamic vinegar, Dijon mustard, and a touch of honey, keeping the carb and calorie content in check.

• The portion size is appropriate for individuals with diabetes, as the salad makes for a nutrient•dense, filling meal.

51. Grilled portobello mushrooms with quinoa

Ingredient:

- 1/2 cup diced tomatoes
- 2 tbsp crumbled feta cheese
- 2 tbsp chopped fresh basil
- 1 tbsp balsamic vinegar
- 1 tsp Dijon mustard

- 4 large portobello mushroom caps, stems removed
- 2 tbsp olive oil, divided
- 1/4 tsp salt
- 1/8 tsp black pepper
- 1 cup cooked quinoa

Instructions:

1. Preheat grill or grill pan to medium•high heat.

2. Brush the portobello mushroom caps with 1 tbsp of the olive oil and season with salt and pepper.

3. Grill the mushrooms for 4•5 minutes per side, until tender and slightly charred.

4. In a medium bowl, combine the cooked quinoa, diced tomatoes, crumbled feta cheese, and chopped fresh basil.

5. In a small bowl, whisk together the remaining 1 tbsp of olive oil, balsamic vinegar, and Dijon mustard to make the dressing.

6. Place the grilled portobello mushroom caps on a serving plate. Spoon the quinoa mixture into the center of each mushroom cap.

7. Drizzle the balsamic dressing over the top of the stuffed mushrooms. Serve immediately.

This grilled portobello mushroom and quinoa dish is diabetic•friendly for the following reasons:

- Portobello mushrooms are a low•carb, high•fiber vegetable that provides essential nutrients.

- Quinoa is a high•fiber, high•protein grain that can help regulate blood sugar levels.

- The addition of diced tomatoes, feta cheese, and fresh basil provides additional vitamins, minerals, and antioxidants without significantly increasing the carb content.

- The balsamic vinegar and Dijon mustard dressing is low in carbs and adds flavor without the need for added sugars.

52. Tomato and cucumber salad with feta and olives

Ingredient:

- 2 cups diced tomatoes
- 1 cup diced cucumber
- 1/4 cup crumbled feta cheese
- 1/4 cup pitted and sliced black olives
- 2 tbsp olive oil
- 1 tbsp red wine vinegar
- 1 tsp dried oregano
- 1/4 tsp salt
- 1/4 tsp black pepper

Instructions:

1. In a large bowl, combine the diced tomatoes, diced cucumber, crumbled feta cheese, and sliced black olives.

2. In a small bowl, whisk together the olive oil, red wine vinegar, dried oregano, salt, and black pepper.

3. Pour the dressing over the salad and toss gently to coat. Serve immediately or refrigerate until ready to serve.

Nutritional Information (per serving):
- Calories: 120
- Total Carbohydrates: 6g
- Fiber: 2g
- Sugars: 4g
- Protein: 4g
- Fat: 10g
- Sodium: 320mg

This salad is a great option for a diabetic diet as it is low in carbohydrates, high in fiber, and provides a good source of healthy fats from the olive oil and feta cheese. The combination of vegetables, protein, and healthy fats can help regulate blood sugar levels and promote overall health for individuals over 50.

53. Turkey chili with kidney beans and bell peppers

Ingredient:

- 1 lb ground turkey
- 1 tbsp olive oil
- 1 onion, diced
- 2 cloves garlic, minced
- 1 red bell pepper, diced
- 1 green bell pepper, diced
- 1 (15 oz) can no•salt•added kidney beans, rinsed and drained
- 1 (15 oz) can no•salt•added diced tomatoes
- 2 tbsp chili powder
- 1 tsp ground cumin
- 1/2 tsp dried oregano
- 1/4 tsp cayenne pepper (optional)
- 1/4 tsp salt
- 1/8 tsp black pepper
- 2 cups low•sodium chicken or vegetable broth

Instructions:

1. In a large pot or Dutch oven, heat the olive oil over medium•high heat.

2. Add the ground turkey and cook, breaking it up with a wooden spoon, until browned, about 5•7 minutes.

3. Add the diced onion and minced garlic. Cook for 2•3 minutes, until the onion is translucent.

4. Stir in the diced red and green bell peppers, kidney beans, diced tomatoes, chili powder, cumin, oregano, cayenne (if using), salt, and black pepper.

5. Pour in the low•sodium broth and bring the mixture to a boil.

6. Reduce the heat to medium•low and let the chili simmer for 20•25 minutes, stirring occasionally, until the flavors have melded and the chili has thickened. Serve hot, garnished with chopped fresh cilantro or green onions, if desired.

This turkey chili is diabetic•friendly for the following reasons:

- Ground turkey is a lean protein that is low in carbs and high in nutrients.
- Kidney beans are a good source of fiber and protein, which can help regulate blood sugar levels.
- Bell peppers provide vitamins, minerals, and antioxidants without adding many carbs.

54. Spinach and feta stuffed chicken breast

Ingredient:
- 4 boneless, skinless chicken breasts
- 1 cup fresh spinach, chopped
- 1/2 cup crumbled feta cheese
- 2 tbsp olive oil
- 1 tsp dried oregano
- 1/4 tsp salt
- 1/4 tsp black pepper

Instructions:
1. Preheat your oven to 375°F (190°C).

2. In a small bowl, mix together the chopped spinach, crumbled feta cheese, 1 tbsp of the olive oil, and 1/2 tsp of the dried oregano.

3. Using a sharp knife, cut a horizontal slit through the thickest part of each chicken breast to create a pocket, being careful not to cut all the way through.

4. Stuff the spinach and feta mixture evenly into the pockets of the chicken breasts.

5. In a small bowl, mix together the remaining 1 tbsp of olive oil, 1/2 tsp of dried oregano, salt, and black pepper. Brush the outside of the chicken breasts with the oil and seasoning mixture.

6. Place the stuffed chicken breasts in a baking dish and bake for 25•30 minutes, or until the chicken is cooked through and the internal temperature reaches 165°F (75°C). Serve the spinach and feta stuffed chicken breasts immediately.

Nutritional Information (per serving):
- Calories: 250
- Total Carbohydrates: 3g
- Fiber: 1g
- Sugars: 1g
- Protein: 32g
- Fat: 13g
- Sodium: 450mg

This dish is a great option for a diabetic diet as it is low in carbohydrates, high in protein, and provides a good source of healthy fats from the olive oil and feta cheese. The spinach also adds fiber and important vitamins and minerals. This recipe is suitable for individuals over 50 who are following a diabetic diet.

55. Butternut squash soup with a dollop of Greek yogurt

Ingredient:

- 1 medium butternut squash, peeled, seeded, and cubed (about 4 cups)
- 1 onion, diced
- 2 cloves garlic, minced
- 4 cups low•sodium chicken or vegetable broth
- 1 tsp ground cumin
- 1/2 tsp ground cinnamon
- 1/4 tsp ground nutmeg
- 1/4 tsp salt
- 1/4 tsp black pepper
- 1/2 cup plain Greek yogurt

Instructions:

1. In a large pot or Dutch oven, sauté the diced onion in a small amount of olive oil over medium heat until translucent, about 5 minutes.

2. Add the minced garlic and sauté for an additional minute.

3. Add the cubed butternut squash, broth, cumin, cinnamon, nutmeg, salt, and pepper. Bring the mixture to a boil.

4. Reduce the heat to low, cover the pot, and simmer for 20•25 minutes, or until the squash is very soft.

5. Using an immersion blender or a regular blender, puree the soup until smooth. Serve the soup warm, with a dollop of plain Greek yogurt on top.

Nutritional Information (per serving):
- Calories: 150
- Total Carbohydrates: 20g
- Fiber: 4g
- Sugars: 6g
- Protein: 6g
- Fat: 5g
- Sodium: 350mg

This butternut squash soup is a great option for a diabetic diet as it is low in carbohydrates, high in fiber, and provides a good source of vitamins and minerals. The addition of the Greek yogurt adds a creamy texture and a boost of protein, making it a satisfying and nutritious meal for individuals over 50 following a diabetic diet.

56. Baked salmon with dill and lemon

Ingredient:
- 4 (4 oz) salmon fillets
- 1 tbsp olive oil
- 2 tbsp chopped fresh dill
- 1 tbsp lemon juice
- 1 tsp grated lemon zest
- 1/4 tsp salt
- 1/8 tsp black pepper

Instructions:
1. Preheat oven to 400°F.

2. Place the salmon fillets on a baking sheet lined with parchment paper.

3. In a small bowl, mix together the olive oil, chopped dill, lemon juice, lemon zest, salt, and black pepper.

4. Spoon the dill•lemon mixture evenly over the top of the salmon fillets.

5. Bake for 12•15 minutes, or until the salmon is opaque and flakes easily with a fork. Serve immediately.

This baked salmon dish is diabetic•friendly for the following reasons:

- Salmon is a lean protein that is high in healthy omega•3 fatty acids, which can help regulate blood sugar levels.

- The dill and lemon flavors add taste without the need for added sugars or sauces.

- The portion size of a 4 oz salmon fillet is appropriate for individuals with diabetes, as it provides a balanced, nutrient•dense meal.

- Baking the salmon is a healthier cooking method compared to frying, as it doesn't require additional oils or fats.

This recipe is easy to prepare and can be a delicious, diabetes•friendly option for a main dish. Serve the baked salmon with a side of steamed vegetables or a small salad for a complete, well•balanced meal. Enjoy!

57. Grilled chicken breast with quinoa and steamed broccoli

Ingredient:

- 4 boneless, skinless chicken breasts
- 1 tbsp olive oil
- 1 tsp dried oregano
- 1/4 tsp salt
- 1/8 tsp black pepper
- 1 cup cooked quinoa
- 4 cups broccoli florets
- 1 tbsp lemon juice
- 1 tsp Dijon mustard
- 1 tsp honey
- 1/4 tsp salt
- 1/8 tsp black pepper

Instructions:

1. Preheat grill or grill pan to medium•high heat.

2. Brush the chicken breasts with olive oil and season with dried oregano, 1/4 tsp of salt, and 1/8 tsp of black pepper.

3. Grill the chicken for 5•7 minutes per side, until cooked through. Allow to rest for 5 minutes, then slice or chop the chicken.

4. While the chicken is grilling, steam the broccoli florets for 5•7 minutes, until tender•crisp.

5. In a small bowl, whisk together the lemon juice, Dijon mustard, honey, 1/4 tsp of salt, and 1/8 tsp of black pepper to make the dressing.

6. Divide the cooked quinoa, grilled chicken, and steamed broccoli evenly among 4 plates. Drizzle the lemon•Dijon dressing over the top of each serving.

This grilled chicken, quinoa, and broccoli dish is diabetic•friendly for the following reasons:

- Grilled chicken is a lean protein that is low in carbs and high in nutrients.

- Quinoa is a high•fiber, high•protein grain that can help regulate blood sugar levels.

- Broccoli is a low•carb, high•fiber vegetable that provides essential vitamins and minerals.

- The lemon•Dijon dressing is made with a small amount of honey, keeping the carb and calorie content in check.

58. Beef stir•fry with mixed vegetables and brown rice

Ingredient:
- 1 lb lean beef sirloin, thinly sliced
- 2 tbsp low•sodium soy sauce
- 1 tbsp rice vinegar
- 1 tsp sesame oil
- 1 tbsp olive oil
- 1/4 tsp salt
- 1/4 tsp black pepper
- 1 tsp grated ginger
- 2 cloves garlic, minced
- 2 cups mixed vegetables (such as broccoli, bell peppers, snow peas, and carrots), chopped
- 1 cup cooked brown rice

Instructions:

1. In a small bowl, combine the soy sauce, rice vinegar, sesame oil, grated ginger, and minced garlic. Add the sliced beef and toss to coat. Let marinate for 15•20 minutes.

2. Heat the olive oil in a large skillet or wok over high heat. Add the marinated beef and stir•fry for 2•3 minutes, until the beef is lightly browned.

3. Add the chopped mixed vegetables to the skillet and continue to stir•fry for 3•4 minutes, until the vegetables are tender•crisp.

4. Stir in the cooked brown rice and season with salt and black pepper. Cook for an additional 1•2 minutes, until the rice is heated through. Serve the beef stir•fry with mixed vegetables and brown rice immediately.

Nutritional Information (per serving):
- Calories: 350
- Total Carbohydrates: 35g
- Fiber: 5g
- Sugars: 4g
- Protein: 30g
- Fat: 12g
- Sodium: 450mg

This beef stir•fry with mixed vegetables and brown rice is a great option for a diabetic diet as it is balanced in carbohydrates, protein, and healthy fats. The lean beef provides a good source of protein, while the mixed vegetables and brown rice offer fiber and important vitamins and minerals. This dish is suitable for individuals over 50 following a diabetic diet.

59. Spaghetti squash with meat sauce

Ingredient:

- 1 tsp dried oregano
- 1 tsp dried basil
- 1/4 tsp red pepper flakes (optional)
- 1/4 tsp salt
- 1/4 tsp black pepper

- 1 medium spaghetti squash, halved lengthwise and seeded
- 1 lb lean ground turkey or ground beef
- 1 onion, diced
- 2 tbsp grated Parmesan cheese (optional)
- 2 cloves garlic, minced
- 1 (14.5 oz) can diced tomatoes
- 1 (6 oz) can tomato paste

Instructions:

1. Preheat your oven to 400°F (200°C).

2. Place the spaghetti squash halves cut-side down on a baking sheet. Bake for 40-50 minutes, or until the squash is tender and easily shreds with a fork.

3. In a large skillet, cook the ground turkey or beef over medium heat, breaking it up as it cooks, until no longer pink, about 5-7 minutes.

4. Add the diced onion and minced garlic to the skillet and cook for an additional 2-3 minutes, until the onion is translucent.

5. Stir in the diced tomatoes, tomato paste, dried oregano, dried basil, red pepper flakes (if using), salt, and black pepper. Simmer the sauce for 10-15 minutes, stirring occasionally, until thickened.

6. Use a fork to shred the cooked spaghetti squash into strands. Serve the spaghetti squash topped with the meat sauce and, if desired, a sprinkle of grated Parmesan cheese.

Nutritional Information (per serving):
- Calories: 250
- Total Carbohydrates: 20g
- Fiber: 5g
- Sugars: 8g
- Protein: 25g
- Fat: 10g
- Sodium: 450mg

This spaghetti squash with meat sauce is a great option for a diabetic diet as it is low in carbohydrates, high in protein, and provides a good source of fiber and important vitamins and minerals. The spaghetti squash serves as a healthier alternative to traditional pasta, making this dish a suitable choice for individuals over 50 following a diabetic diet.

60. Grilled shrimp with garlic and zucchini noodles

Ingredient:
- 1 lb large shrimp, peeled and deveined
- 3 cloves garlic, minced
- 2 tbsp olive oil, divided
- 1/4 tsp salt
- 1/4 tsp black pepper
- 3 medium zucchini, spiralized or julienned into noodles
- 1 tbsp lemon juice
- 2 tbsp chopped fresh parsley

Instructions:

1. In a medium bowl, combine the shrimp, minced garlic, 1 tbsp of the olive oil, salt, and black pepper. Toss to coat the shrimp evenly.

2. Preheat your grill or grill pan to medium•high heat.

3. Thread the seasoned shrimp onto skewers (if using wooden skewers, soak them in water for 30 minutes beforehand to prevent burning).

4. Grill the shrimp for 2•3 minutes per side, or until they are opaque and cooked through.

5. In a large skillet, heat the remaining 1 tbsp of olive oil over medium heat. Add the spiralized or julienned zucchini noodles and sauté for 2•3 minutes, just until they start to soften.

6. Remove the skillet from the heat and stir in the lemon juice and chopped parsley. Serve the grilled shrimp over the garlic zucchini noodles.

Nutritional Information (per serving):
- Calories: 200
- Total Carbohydrates: 8g
- Fiber: 2g
- Sugars: 4g
- Protein: 22g
- Fat: 10g
- Sodium: 350mg

This grilled shrimp with garlic and zucchini noodles is a great option for a diabetic diet as it is low in carbohydrates, high in protein, and provides a good source of healthy fats from the olive oil. The zucchini noodles serve as a low•carb alternative to traditional pasta, making this dish suitable for individuals over 50 following a diabetic diet.

61. Herb•crusted pork tenderloin with roasted Brussels sprouts

Ingredient:

- 1 lb pork tenderloin
- 2 tbsp Dijon mustard
- 1 tbsp chopped fresh rosemary
- 1 tbsp chopped fresh thyme
- 1 tbsp olive oil
- 1/4 tsp salt
- 1/4 tsp black pepper
- 1 lb Brussels sprouts, trimmed and halved
- 1 tbsp olive oil
- 1/4 tsp salt
- 1/4 tsp black pepper

Instructions:

1. Preheat your oven to 400°F (200°C).

2. In a small bowl, mix together the Dijon mustard, chopped rosemary, chopped thyme, 1 tbsp of olive oil, salt, and black pepper.

3. Rub the herb•mustard mixture all over the pork tenderloin.

4. Place the pork tenderloin on a baking sheet or in a roasting pan.

5. In a separate bowl, toss the trimmed and halved Brussels sprouts with 1 tbsp of olive oil, salt, and black pepper.

6. Arrange the Brussels sprouts around the pork tenderloin on the baking sheet or in the roasting pan.

7. Roast the pork tenderloin and Brussels sprouts in the preheated oven for 25•30 minutes, or until the pork reaches an internal temperature of 145°F (63°C) and the Brussels sprouts are tender and lightly browned.

8. Let the pork tenderloin rest for 5 minutes before slicing and serving. Serve the sliced pork tenderloin with the roasted Brussels sprouts.

This herb•crusted pork tenderloin with roasted Brussels sprouts is a great option for a diabetic diet as it is low in carbohydrates, high in protein, and provides a good source of fiber and important vitamins and minerals. The combination of the flavorful pork and the roasted Brussels sprouts makes for a satisfying and nutritious meal for individuals over 50 following a diabetic diet.

62. Chicken and vegetable kebabs with a side salad

Ingredient:

Kebabs:
• 1 lb boneless, skinless chicken breasts, cut into 1•inch cubes
• 1 red bell pepper, cut into 1•inch pieces
• 1 zucchini, cut into 1•inch pieces
• 1 red onion, cut into 1•inch pieces
• 2 tbsp olive oil
• 1 tsp dried oregano
• 1/4 tsp salt
• 1/4 tsp black pepper

Side Salad:
• 5 cups mixed greens (such as spinach, arugula, and romaine)
• 1 cucumber, sliced
• 1 tomato, diced
• 2 tbsp balsamic vinegar
• 1 tbsp olive oil
• 1/4 tsp salt
• 1/4 tsp black pepper

Instructions:

1. Preheat your grill or grill pan to medium•high heat.

2. In a large bowl, combine the cubed chicken, bell pepper, zucchini, and red onion. Drizzle with 2 tbsp of olive oil and sprinkle with dried oregano, salt, and black pepper. Toss to coat the ingredients evenly.

3. Thread the chicken and vegetables onto skewers, alternating the ingredients.

4. Grill the kebabs for 12•15 minutes, turning occasionally, until the chicken is cooked through and the vegetables are tender.

5. In a large salad bowl, combine the mixed greens, sliced cucumber, and diced tomato.

6. In a small bowl, whisk together the balsamic vinegar, 1 tbsp of olive oil, salt, and black pepper.

7. Drizzle the dressing over the salad and toss to coat. Serve the grilled chicken and vegetable kebabs with the side salad.

This chicken and vegetable kebab dish with a side salad is a great option for a diabetic diet as it is balanced in carbohydrates, protein, and healthy fats. The grilled chicken and vegetables provide a good source of lean protein and fiber, while the side salad adds additional nutrients and fiber. This meal is suitable for individuals over 50 following a diabetic diet.

63. Baked cod with a side of sautéed spinach

Ingredient:

Baked Cod:
- 4 (6 oz) cod fillets
- 2 tbsp olive oil
- 1 tsp paprika
- 1/4 tsp salt
- 1/4 tsp black pepper

Sautéed Spinach:
- 1 tbsp olive oil
- 4 cups fresh spinach, washed and stems removed
- 2 cloves garlic, minced
- 1/4 tsp salt
- 1/4 tsp black pepper

Instructions:

Baked Cod:
1. Preheat your oven to 400°F (200°C).

2. Place the cod fillets in a baking dish and drizzle with 2 tbsp of olive oil. Sprinkle the paprika, salt, and black pepper over the top.

3. Bake the cod for 15•20 minutes, or until it flakes easily with a fork and reaches an internal temperature of 145°F (63°C).

Sautéed Spinach:
1. In a large skillet, heat 1 tbsp of olive oil over medium heat.

2. Add the fresh spinach and sauté for 2•3 minutes, until the spinach is wilted.

3. Add the minced garlic, salt, and black pepper. Sauté for an additional 1•2 minutes, until the garlic is fragrant.

Serving: Serve the baked cod fillets with the sautéed spinach on the side.

This baked cod with sautéed spinach is a great option for a diabetic diet as it is low in carbohydrates, high in protein, and provides a good source of healthy fats from the olive oil. The cod is a lean protein source, while the spinach adds fiber and important vitamins and minerals. This dish is suitable for individuals over 50 following a diabetic diet.

64. Turkey meatloaf with mashed cauliflower

Ingredient:

Turkey Meatloaf:
• 1 lb ground turkey
• 1/2 cup whole wheat breadcrumbs
• 1/4 cup diced onion
• 1 clove garlic, minced
• 1 egg, lightly beaten
• 2 tbsp tomato paste
• 1 tsp dried oregano
• 1/4 tsp salt
• 1/4 tsp black pepper

Mashed Cauliflower:
• 1 head of cauliflower, cut into florets
• 2 tbsp unsweetened almond milk
• 1 tbsp olive oil
• 1/4 tsp salt
• 1/4 tsp black pepper

Instructions:

Turkey Meatloaf:

1. Preheat your oven to 375°F (190°C).

2. In a large bowl, combine the ground turkey, breadcrumbs, diced onion, minced garlic, egg, tomato paste, dried oregano, salt, and black pepper. Mix until well combined.

3. Transfer the turkey mixture to a loaf pan and shape it into a loaf.

4. Bake the meatloaf for 45•50 minutes, or until it reaches an internal temperature of 165°F (75°C). Let the meatloaf rest for 5 minutes before slicing and serving.

Mashed Cauliflower:

1. In a large pot, bring a few inches of water to a boil. Add the cauliflower florets and steam for 10•12 minutes, or until the cauliflower is very tender.

2. Drain the cauliflower and transfer it to a food processor or blender.

3. Add the unsweetened almond milk, olive oil, salt, and black pepper. Blend or process until the cauliflower is smooth and creamy. Serve the mashed cauliflower alongside the sliced turkey meatloaf.

This turkey meatloaf with mashed cauliflower is a great option for a diabetic diet as it is low in carbohydrates, high in protein, and provides a good source of fiber and important vitamins and minerals. The mashed cauliflower serves as a low•carb alternative to traditional mashed potatoes, making this dish suitable for individuals over 50 following a diabetic diet.

65. Stuffed cabbage rolls
with lean ground beef and brown rice

Ingredient:

- 1 medium head of green cabbage
- 1 lb lean ground beef
- 1 cup cooked brown rice
- 1 onion, finely chopped
- 2 cloves garlic, minced
- 1 (14.5 oz) can diced tomatoes
- 2 tbsp tomato paste
- 1 tsp dried oregano
- 1/4 tsp salt
- 1/4 tsp black pepper

Instructions:

1. Bring a large pot of water to a boil. Carefully add the whole head of cabbage and cook for 5•7 minutes, or until the outer leaves are softened. Remove the cabbage from the water and let it cool slightly.

2. Carefully peel off the softened cabbage leaves, one at a time, and set them aside. You should have about 12•14 leaves.

3. In a large bowl, combine the lean ground beef, cooked brown rice, chopped onion, minced garlic, diced tomatoes, tomato paste, dried oregano, salt, and black pepper. Mix well until the ingredients are evenly distributed.

4. Place about 1/4 cup of the beef and rice mixture onto the center of each cabbage leaf. Fold the sides of the leaf over the filling and then roll up the leaf tightly to enclose the filling.

5. Arrange the stuffed cabbage rolls seam•side down in a baking dish.

6. Cover the dish with foil and bake at 375°F (190°C) for 45•55 minutes, or until the cabbage rolls are heated through and the filling is cooked.Serve the stuffed cabbage rolls warm.

This stuffed cabbage rolls dish is a great option for a diabetic diet as it is balanced in carbohydrates, protein, and fiber. The lean ground beef and brown rice provide a good source of protein and complex carbohydrates, while the cabbage adds fiber and important vitamins and minerals. This recipe is suitable for individuals over 50 following a diabetic diet.

66. Lemon and herb roasted chicken with green beans

Ingredient:
- 1 whole chicken, 3•4 lbs
- 2 tbsp olive oil
- 2 tbsp lemon juice
- 2 tsp dried thyme
- 2 tsp dried rosemary
- 1 tsp garlic powder
- 1 tsp salt
- 1/2 tsp black pepper
- 1 lb green beans, trimmed

Instructions:

1. Preheat oven to 400°F.

2. In a small bowl, mix together the olive oil, lemon juice, thyme, rosemary, garlic powder, salt, and pepper.

3. Pat the chicken dry with paper towels and place it in a large roasting pan. Rub the lemon•herb mixture all over the chicken, making sure to get it under the skin as well.

4. Arrange the green beans around the chicken in the roasting pan.

5. Roast the chicken and green beans for 60•75 minutes, or until the chicken is cooked through (internal temperature reaches 165°F) and the green beans are tender.

6. Let the chicken rest for 10 minutes before carving and serving.

Nutritional Information (per serving, assuming 4 servings):
- Calories: 350
- Total Carbs: 12g
- Fiber: 4g
- Net Carbs: 8g
- Protein: 40g
- Fat: 18g

This recipe is diabetic•friendly, as it is low in carbs and high in protein and healthy fats. The lemon and herbs add flavor without the need for excessive salt or sugar. The green beans provide fiber and additional nutrients. Enjoy this delicious and nutritious meal!

67. Lentil and vegetable stew

Ingredient:

- 1 cup dry brown or green lentils, rinsed
- 4 cups low•sodium vegetable broth
- 1 tbsp olive oil
- 1 onion, diced
- 3 cloves garlic, minced
- 2 carrots, peeled and diced
- 2 celery stalks, diced
- 1 zucchini, diced
- 1 (14.5 oz) can diced tomatoes, no salt added
- 2 tsp dried thyme
- 1 tsp dried oregano
- 1/2 tsp smoked paprika
- Salt and black pepper to taste
- Fresh parsley, chopped (for garnish)

Instructions:

1. In a large pot, combine the lentils and vegetable broth. Bring to a boil, then reduce heat and simmer for 15•20 minutes, until lentils are tender.

2. In a separate large pot or Dutch oven, heat the olive oil over medium heat. Add the onion and garlic, and sauté for 2•3 minutes until fragrant.

3. Add the carrots, celery, and zucchini to the pot. Cook for 5•7 minutes, stirring occasionally, until vegetables are starting to soften.

4. Stir in the diced tomatoes, thyme, oregano, and smoked paprika. Season with salt and pepper to taste.

5. Add the cooked lentils and their broth to the vegetable mixture. Bring the stew to a simmer and let it cook for 10•15 minutes, allowing the flavors to meld. Serve the lentil and vegetable stew hot, garnished with fresh chopped parsley.

This lentil and vegetable stew is a great diabetic•friendly option, as it is high in fiber, protein, and complex carbohydrates, while being low in fat and calories. The variety of vegetables provides a range of essential vitamins and minerals. Enjoy this hearty and nutritious stew!

68. Eggplant lasagna with ground turkey

Ingredient:

- 1 tsp dried basil
- 1/2 tsp red pepper flakes (optional)
- Salt and black pepper to taste
- 1 cup part•skim ricotta cheese
- 1 cup shredded part•skim mozzarella cheese
- 1/4 cup grated Parmesan cheese
- 2 tbsp chopped fresh parsley
- 2 medium eggplants, sliced lengthwise into 1/4•inch thick slices
- 1 lb ground turkey
- 1 onion, diced
- 3 cloves garlic, minced
- 1 (28 oz) can crushed tomatoes, no salt added
- 2 tsp dried oregano

Instructions:

1. Preheat oven to 375°F.

2. Arrange the eggplant slices in a single layer on a baking sheet. Bake for 15•20 minutes, flipping halfway, until eggplant is tender and lightly browned. Set aside.

3. In a large skillet, cook the ground turkey over medium heat, breaking it up as it cooks, until no longer pink, about 5•7 minutes. Add the onion and garlic, and cook for an additional 2•3 minutes until fragrant.

4. Stir in the crushed tomatoes, oregano, basil, and red pepper flakes (if using). Season with salt and pepper to taste. Simmer for 10 minutes.

5. In a small bowl, mix together the ricotta, 1/2 cup of the mozzarella, and the Parmesan cheese.

6. Spread a thin layer of the turkey•tomato sauce in the bottom of a 9x13•inch baking dish. Arrange a layer of the roasted eggplant slices over the sauce. Spread half of the ricotta cheese mixture over the eggplant, then top with another layer of eggplant slices.

7. Pour the remaining turkey•tomato sauce over the eggplant and spread evenly. Top with the remaining mozzarella cheese.

8. Bake for 30•35 minutes, until the cheese is melted and bubbly. Let stand for 5 minutes before serving. Garnish with chopped fresh parsley.

This eggplant lasagna is a delicious and diabetic•friendly option, as it is low in carbs and high in protein and fiber. The use of ground turkey instead of beef helps keep the fat content down, while the eggplant provides a satisfying, low•carb alternative to traditional pasta.

69. Grilled tofu with a side of quinoa and steamed broccoli

Ingredient:

Tofu:
- 1 block (14 oz) extra•firm tofu, drained and cut into 1/2•inch thick slices
- 2 tbsp low•sodium soy sauce or tamari
- 1 tbsp rice vinegar
- 1 tsp sesame oil
- 1 tsp honey
- 1 tsp grated ginger
- 1/4 tsp red pepper flakes (optional)

Quinoa:
- 1 cup uncooked quinoa, rinsed
- 2 cups low•sodium vegetable or chicken broth

Broccoli: 1 lb broccoli florets

Instructions:

1. Preheat grill or grill pan to medium•high heat.

2. In a shallow dish, whisk together the soy sauce, rice vinegar, sesame oil, honey, ginger, and red pepper flakes (if using). Add the tofu slices and gently toss to coat. Let marinate for 10•15 minutes.

3. In a medium saucepan, combine the quinoa and broth. Bring to a boil, then reduce heat to low, cover, and simmer for 15•20 minutes, until quinoa is tender and liquid is absorbed.

4. While the quinoa is cooking, steam the broccoli florets until tender•crisp, about 5•7 minutes.

5. Grill the marinated tofu slices for 3•4 minutes per side, or until lightly charred and heated through.

6. Serve the grilled tofu over the cooked quinoa, with the steamed broccoli on the side. Drizzle any remaining marinade over the tofu, if desired.

This grilled tofu dish is a great diabetic•friendly option, as it is high in protein, fiber, and complex carbohydrates, while being low in fat and calories. The quinoa and broccoli provide additional nutrients and fiber to help manage blood sugar levels. Enjoy this balanced and flavorful meal!

70. Cauliflower crust pizza with vegetables and low•fat cheese

Ingredient:

Toppings:
• 1 cup no•sugar•added marinara sauce
• 1 cup shredded part•skim mozzarella cheese
• 1/2 cup sliced mushrooms
• 1/2 cup diced bell peppers
• 1/4 cup sliced black olives
• 2 tbsp chopped fresh basil (optional)

Cauliflower Crust:
• 4 cups riced cauliflower (about 1 medium head)
• 1 egg, beaten
• 1/2 cup grated Parmesan cheese
• 1/2 tsp dried oregano
• 1/4 tsp garlic powder
• 1/4 tsp salt

Instructions:

1. Preheat oven to 400°F. Line a baking sheet with parchment paper.

2. To make the cauliflower crust, place the riced cauliflower in a microwave•safe bowl and microwave for 5•7 minutes, until tender. Allow to cool slightly, then transfer to a clean kitchen towel or cheesecloth and squeeze out as much moisture as possible.

3. In a medium bowl, mix the squeezed cauliflower, egg, Parmesan, oregano, garlic powder, and salt until well combined.

4. Press the cauliflower mixture onto the prepared baking sheet, forming a thin, even crust.

5. Bake the crust for 20•25 minutes, until golden brown and crispy.

6. Remove the crust from the oven and top with the marinara sauce, mozzarella cheese, mushrooms, bell peppers, and black olives.

7. Return the pizza to the oven and bake for an additional 10•15 minutes, until the cheese is melted and bubbly.

8. Remove the pizza from the oven and let it cool for a few minutes. Garnish with fresh basil, if desired. Slice and serve.

This cauliflower crust pizza is a great diabetic•friendly option, as it is low in carbs and high in protein and fiber. The use of low•fat cheese and a variety of vegetables provides additional nutrients and helps keep the overall calorie and fat content in check. Enjoy this delicious and healthy pizza!

71. Baked halibut with a side of asparagus

Ingredient:

- 4 (6 oz) halibut fillets
- 2 tbsp olive oil
- 1 tsp lemon zest
- 2 tbsp lemon juice
- 2 tsp Dijon mustard
- 1 tsp dried dill
- 1/4 tsp salt
- 1/4 tsp black pepper
- 1 lb asparagus, trimmed
- 1 tbsp unsalted butter, melted

Instructions:

1. Preheat oven to 400°F. Lightly grease a baking sheet or oven•safe dish.

2. In a small bowl, whisk together the olive oil, lemon zest, lemon juice, Dijon mustard, dried dill, salt, and black pepper.

3. Place the halibut fillets on the prepared baking sheet or dish. Spoon the lemon•herb mixture over the top of the fish, making sure to evenly coat each fillet.

4. Arrange the asparagus spears around the halibut. Drizzle the melted butter over the asparagus.

5. Bake for 15•20 minutes, or until the halibut is opaque and flakes easily with a fork, and the asparagus is tender•crisp.

6. Serve the baked halibut immediately, with the roasted asparagus on the side.

This baked halibut with asparagus dish is an excellent choice for a diabetic•friendly, over 50 diet. Halibut is a lean, high•protein fish that is low in carbs and calories. The asparagus provides fiber, vitamins, and minerals, while the lemon•herb seasoning adds flavor without the need for excessive salt or sugar. This meal is well•balanced and supports healthy blood sugar management.

72. Chicken fajitas with bell peppers and whole grain tortillas

Ingredient:

- 1 lb boneless, skinless chicken breasts, sliced into thin strips
- 2 tbsp olive oil
- 1 tbsp chili powder
- 1 tsp ground cumin
- 1 tsp garlic powder
- 1/2 tsp smoked paprika
- 1/4 tsp salt
- 1/4 tsp black pepper
- 2 bell peppers, sliced into thin strips
- 1 onion, sliced
- 8 whole grain tortillas (6•inch size)
- Toppings (optional): diced avocado, salsa, plain Greek yogurt, shredded lettuce

Instructions:

1. In a large bowl, combine the chicken strips, 1 tbsp olive oil, chili powder, cumin, garlic powder, smoked paprika, salt, and black pepper. Toss to coat the chicken evenly.

2. Heat the remaining 1 tbsp of olive oil in a large skillet or grill pan over medium•high heat. Add the chicken and cook for 5•7 minutes, stirring occasionally, until the chicken is cooked through and no longer pink.

3. Add the sliced bell peppers and onion to the skillet. Cook for an additional 5•7 minutes, stirring occasionally, until the vegetables are tender•crisp.

4. Warm the whole grain tortillas according to package instructions.

5. Serve the chicken and vegetable mixture in the warm tortillas. Top with your desired toppings, such as diced avocado, salsa, plain Greek yogurt, and shredded lettuce.

This chicken fajita dish is a great diabetic•friendly option for individuals over 50. The use of whole grain tortillas, lean chicken, and a variety of fresh vegetables provides a balanced meal that is high in protein, fiber, and complex carbohydrates, while being low in fat and calories. The spices add flavor without the need for excessive salt or sugar. Enjoy this delicious and nutritious fajita meal!

73. Mushroom and barley risotto

Ingredient:

- 1 cup uncooked pearl barley
- 4 cups low•sodium vegetable or chicken broth
- 1 tbsp olive oil
- 1 onion, diced
- 8 oz sliced mushrooms (such as cremini or button)
- 3 cloves garlic, minced
- 1 tsp dried thyme
- 1/4 tsp salt
- 1/4 tsp black pepper
- 1/4 cup grated Parmesan cheese
- 2 tbsp chopped fresh parsley (optional)

Instructions:

1. In a medium saucepan, bring the broth to a simmer over medium heat. Reduce heat to low and keep the broth warm.

2. In a large skillet, heat the olive oil over medium heat. Add the onion and sauté for 3•4 minutes until translucent.

3. Add the sliced mushrooms and continue cooking for 5•7 minutes, stirring occasionally, until the mushrooms are tender and lightly browned.

4. Stir in the garlic and thyme, and cook for an additional minute until fragrant.

5. Add the uncooked barley to the skillet and stir to coat the grains with the oil and vegetable mixture.

6. Ladle in 1/2 cup of the warm broth and stir constantly until the liquid is absorbed, about 5 minutes. Continue adding the broth, 1/2 cup at a time, stirring constantly, until the barley is tender and has a creamy texture, about 25•30 minutes total.

7. Remove the risotto from heat and stir in the salt, black pepper, and Parmesan cheese. Serve the mushroom and barley risotto warm, garnished with chopped fresh parsley, if desired.

This mushroom and barley risotto is a diabetic•friendly, over 50 dish that is high in fiber, complex carbohydrates, and nutrients. The use of barley instead of traditional arborio rice helps keep the carb and calorie content in check, while the mushrooms and Parmesan cheese provide a savory, satisfying flavor. Enjoy this creamy and comforting risotto as part of a balanced diabetic•friendly meal.

74. Roasted chicken thighs with a side of roasted carrots

Ingredient:

• 8 bone•in, skin•on chicken thighs
• 2 tbsp olive oil, divided
• 1 tsp dried thyme
• 1 tsp garlic powder
• 1/2 tsp salt
• 1/4 tsp black pepper
• 1 lb carrots, peeled and cut into 1•inch pieces
• 1 tbsp chopped fresh parsley (optional)

Instructions:

1. Preheat oven to 400°F. Line a large baking sheet with parchment paper or foil.

2. In a large bowl, combine the chicken thighs, 1 tbsp of the olive oil, thyme, garlic powder, salt, and black pepper. Toss to coat the chicken evenly.

3. Arrange the chicken thighs, skin•side up, on the prepared baking sheet.

4. In the same bowl, toss the carrot pieces with the remaining 1 tbsp of olive oil.

5. Arrange the carrots around the chicken thighs on the baking sheet, making sure they are in a single layer.

6. Roast the chicken and carrots for 35•40 minutes, or until the chicken is cooked through (internal temperature reaches 165°F) and the carrots are tender.

7. Remove the baking sheet from the oven and let the chicken rest for 5 minutes.

8. Serve the roasted chicken thighs with the roasted carrots. Garnish with chopped fresh parsley, if desired.

This roasted chicken and carrots dish is an excellent choice for a diabetic•friendly, over 50 diet. Chicken thighs are a flavorful, high•protein option, and the roasted carrots provide fiber, vitamins, and minerals. The simple seasoning adds flavor without the need for excessive salt or sugar. This meal is well•balanced and supports healthy blood sugar management.

75. Moroccan chicken with chickpeas and spinach

Ingredient:

- 1 lb boneless, skinless chicken breasts, cut into 1•inch pieces
- 1 tbsp olive oil
- 1 onion, diced
- 3 cloves garlic, minced
- 1 tbsp grated fresh ginger
- 1 tsp ground cumin
- 1 tsp paprika
- 1/2 tsp ground cinnamon
- 1/4 tsp cayenne pepper (optional)
- 1 (15 oz) can no•salt•added chickpeas, rinsed and drained
- 1 (14.5 oz) can no•salt•added diced tomatoes
- 1 cup low•sodium chicken broth
- 4 cups fresh spinach, roughly chopped
- 2 tbsp chopped fresh cilantro
- Salt and black pepper to taste

Instructions:

1. In a large skillet or Dutch oven, heat the olive oil over medium•high heat.

2. Add the chicken pieces and cook for 3•4 minutes, until lightly browned on the outside. Transfer the chicken to a plate and set aside.

3. Reduce the heat to medium and add the onion to the skillet. Cook for 5•7 minutes, stirring occasionally, until the onion is softened.

4. Stir in the garlic, ginger, cumin, paprika, cinnamon, and cayenne (if using). Cook for 1 minute, until fragrant.

5. Add the chickpeas, diced tomatoes, and chicken broth to the skillet. Bring the mixture to a simmer.

6. Return the cooked chicken to the skillet and simmer for 10•15 minutes, until the chicken is cooked through and the sauce has thickened slightly. Stir in the chopped spinach and cook for 2•3 minutes, until the spinach is wilted.

7. Remove the skillet from heat and stir in the chopped cilantro. Season with salt and black pepper to taste. Serve the Moroccan chicken and chickpea mixture warm.

This Moroccan•inspired chicken dish is a great diabetic•friendly option for individuals over 50. The combination of lean chicken, fiber•rich chickpeas, and nutrient•dense spinach provides a well•balanced meal that is high in protein, fiber, and complex carbohydrates, while being low in fat and calories. The warm spices add flavor without the need for excessive salt or sugar.

76. Beef and vegetable kebabs

Ingredient:

- 1 lb beef sirloin or flank steak, cut into 1•inch cubes
- 1 red bell pepper, cut into 1•inch pieces
- 1 yellow bell pepper, cut into 1•inch pieces
- 1 red onion, cut into 1•inch pieces
- 8 oz mushrooms, halved
- 2 tbsp olive oil
- 2 tbsp balsamic vinegar
- 1 tsp dried oregano
- 1/2 tsp garlic powder
- 1/4 tsp salt
- 1/4 tsp black pepper

Instructions:

1. Preheat grill or grill pan to medium•high heat.

2. In a large bowl, combine the beef cubes, bell pepper pieces, onion pieces, and mushrooms.

3. In a small bowl, whisk together the olive oil, balsamic vinegar, oregano, garlic powder, salt, and black pepper.

4. Pour the marinade over the beef and vegetables, and toss to coat everything evenly.

5. Thread the marinated beef and vegetables onto skewers, alternating the ingredients.

6. Grill the kebabs for 12•15 minutes, turning occasionally, until the beef is cooked through and the vegetables are tender.

7. Serve the grilled beef and vegetable kebabs immediately.

This beef and vegetable kebab recipe is an excellent choice for a diabetic•friendly, over 50 diet. The lean beef provides a good source of protein, while the variety of vegetables add fiber, vitamins, and minerals. The marinade adds flavor without the need for excessive salt or sugar. Grilling the kebabs is a healthy cooking method that helps retain the nutrients and keeps the dish low in calories and fat. Enjoy this balanced and delicious meal!

77. Vegetarian stuffed peppers with quinoa and black beans

Ingredient:

• 4 large bell peppers (any color), halved lengthwise and seeds removed
• 1 cup cooked quinoa
• 1 (15 oz) can no•salt•added black beans, rinsed and drained
• 1 cup diced tomatoes (fresh or canned, no salt added)
• 1/2 cup frozen corn kernels
• 1/2 cup shredded low•fat cheddar cheese
• 2 tbsp chopped fresh cilantro
• 1 tsp ground cumin
• 1/2 tsp garlic powder
• 1/4 tsp chili powder
• Salt and black pepper to taste

Instructions:

1. Preheat oven to 375°F. Lightly grease a baking dish or line it with parchment paper.

2. Arrange the bell pepper halves, cut•side up, in the prepared baking dish.

3. In a medium bowl, combine the cooked quinoa, black beans, diced tomatoes, corn, cheddar cheese, cilantro, cumin, garlic powder, and chili powder. Season with salt and black pepper to taste.

4. Spoon the quinoa and black bean mixture evenly into the bell pepper halves.

5. Cover the baking dish with foil and bake for 30 minutes.

6. Remove the foil and bake for an additional 10•15 minutes, or until the peppers are tender and the filling is heated through.

7. Serve the stuffed peppers warm.

This vegetarian stuffed pepper dish is an excellent choice for a diabetic•friendly, over 50 diet. The combination of quinoa, black beans, and vegetables provides a good source of fiber, complex carbohydrates, and plant•based protein, while the low•fat cheese adds a touch of creaminess. The simple seasoning adds flavor without the need for excessive salt or sugar. This meal is well•balanced and supports healthy blood sugar management.

78. Shrimp scampi with zucchini noodles

Ingredient:

• 1 lb large shrimp, peeled and deveined
• 2 tbsp olive oil
• 3 cloves garlic, minced
• 1/4 cup dry white wine (or low•sodium chicken broth)
• 2 tbsp fresh lemon juice
• 2 tbsp unsalted butter
• 1/4 cup chopped fresh parsley
• 1/4 tsp red pepper flakes (optional)
• Salt and black pepper to taste
• 3 medium zucchini, spiralized or julienned into noodles

Instructions:

1. In a large skillet, heat the olive oil over medium•high heat.

2. Add the shrimp and garlic to the skillet. Cook for 2•3 minutes, stirring frequently, until the shrimp are starting to turn pink.

3. Pour in the white wine (or chicken broth) and lemon juice. Bring the mixture to a simmer and cook for 2•3 minutes, until the shrimp are cooked through and opaque.

4. Remove the skillet from heat and stir in the butter until melted and well combined.

5. Stir in the chopped parsley and red pepper flakes (if using). Season with salt and black pepper to taste.

6. Add the spiralized or julienned zucchini noodles to the skillet and toss to coat with the shrimp scampi sauce.

7. Serve the shrimp scampi with zucchini noodles immediately.

This shrimp scampi with zucchini noodles dish is an excellent choice for a diabetic•friendly, over 50 diet. The use of zucchini noodles instead of traditional pasta keeps the carb and calorie content low, while the shrimp provides a good source of lean protein. The garlic, lemon, and white wine sauce adds flavor without the need for excessive salt or sugar. This meal is well•balanced and supports healthy blood sugar management.

79. Grilled lamb chops with a side of grilled vegetables

Ingredient:

Lamb Chops:
• 4 (4 oz) lamb loin chops
• 1 tbsp olive oil
• 1 tsp dried rosemary
• 1/2 tsp garlic powder
• 1/4 tsp salt
• 1/4 tsp black pepper

Grilled Vegetables:
• 1 zucchini, sliced into 1/2•inch thick rounds
• 1 yellow squash, sliced into 1/2•inch thick rounds
• 1 red bell pepper, cut into 1•inch pieces
• 1 red onion, cut into 1•inch wedges
• 2 tbsp olive oil
• 1/4 tsp salt
• 1/4 tsp black pepper

Instructions:

1. Preheat grill or grill pan to medium•high heat.

2. In a small bowl, combine the 1 tbsp olive oil, rosemary, garlic powder, 1/4 tsp salt, and 1/4 tsp black pepper. Rub the mixture evenly over the lamb chops.

3. In a large bowl, toss the zucchini, yellow squash, bell pepper, and onion with the 2 tbsp olive oil, 1/4 tsp salt, and 1/4 tsp black pepper.

4. Grill the lamb chops for 3•4 minutes per side, or until they reach the desired doneness (medium•rare to medium).

5. Grill the seasoned vegetables for 5•7 minutes, turning occasionally, until they are tender and lightly charred. Serve the grilled lamb chops with the grilled vegetables.

This grilled lamb chops with grilled vegetables dish is an excellent choice for a diabetic•friendly, over 50 diet. Lamb is a lean, high•protein meat that is low in carbs and calories. The variety of grilled vegetables provides fiber, vitamins, and minerals. The simple seasoning adds flavor without the need for excessive salt or sugar. This meal is well•balanced and supports healthy blood sugar management.

80. Cauliflower and chickpea curry with brown rice

Ingredient:

Curry:
• 1 tbsp olive oil
• 1 onion, diced
• 3 cloves garlic, minced
• 1 tbsp grated fresh ginger
• 2 tsp curry powder
• 1 tsp ground cumin
• 1/2 tsp ground coriander
• 1/4 tsp cayenne pepper (optional)
• 1 (15 oz) can no•salt•added chickpeas, rinsed and drained
• 1 head cauliflower, cut into florets
• 1 (14 oz) can no•salt•added diced tomatoes
• 1 cup low•sodium vegetable broth
• 1/4 cup unsweetened coconut milk
• 2 tbsp chopped fresh cilantro

Brown Rice:
• 1 cup uncooked brown rice
• 2 cups low•sodium vegetable or chicken broth

Instructions:

1. In a large skillet or Dutch oven, heat the olive oil over medium heat.

2. Add the onion and sauté for 3•4 minutes, until translucent.

3. Stir in the garlic, ginger, curry powder, cumin, coriander, and cayenne (if using). Cook for 1 minute, until fragrant.

4. Add the chickpeas, cauliflower florets, diced tomatoes, vegetable broth, and coconut milk. Bring the mixture to a simmer.

5. Reduce heat to low, cover, and let the curry simmer for 20•25 minutes, stirring occasionally, until the cauliflower is tender.

6. While the curry is simmering, prepare the brown rice. In a medium saucepan, combine the brown rice and 2 cups of broth. Bring to a boil, then reduce heat to low, cover, and simmer for 20•25 minutes, until the rice is tender and the liquid is absorbed.

7. Stir the chopped cilantro into the cauliflower and chickpea curry. Serve the curry over the cooked brown rice.

This cauliflower and chickpea curry with brown rice is an excellent choice for a diabetic•friendly, over 50 diet. The combination of vegetables, legumes, and whole grain rice provides a good balance of fiber, complex carbohydrates, and plant•based protein. The spices add flavor without the need for excessive salt or sugar. This meal is well•balanced and supports healthy blood sugar management.

81. Seared scallops with a side of sautéed kale

Ingredient:

Scallops:
- 1 lb sea scallops, patted dry
- 1 tbsp olive oil
- 1/4 tsp salt
- 1/4 tsp black pepper

Kale:
- 1 lb kale, stems removed and leaves chopped
- 1 tbsp olive oil
- 2 cloves garlic, minced
- 1/4 tsp red pepper flakes (optional)
- 1/4 tsp salt
- 1/4 tsp black pepper

Instructions:

1. Heat a large skillet over high heat. Add the 1 tbsp olive oil.

2. Pat the scallops dry with paper towels and season with the 1/4 tsp salt and 1/4 tsp black pepper.

3. Carefully add the scallops to the hot skillet and sear for 2•3 minutes per side, until a golden•brown crust forms and the scallops are opaque in the center. Transfer the seared scallops to a plate and set aside.

4. In the same skillet, heat the 1 tbsp olive oil over medium heat.

5. Add the chopped kale, garlic, red pepper flakes (if using), 1/4 tsp salt, and 1/4 tsp black pepper. Sauté for 5•7 minutes, stirring occasionally, until the kale is wilted and tender.

6. Serve the seared scallops immediately, with the sautéed kale on the side.

This seared scallops with sautéed kale dish is an excellent choice for a diabetic•friendly, over 50 diet. Scallops are a lean, high•protein seafood that is low in carbs and calories. The kale provides fiber, vitamins, and minerals. The simple seasoning adds flavor without the need for excessive salt or sugar. This meal is well•balanced and supports healthy blood sugar management.

82. Stuffed portobello mushrooms with ground turkey

Ingredient:

• 4 large portobello mushroom caps, stems removed and chopped
• 1 lb ground turkey
• 1 small onion, diced
• 2 cloves garlic, minced
• 1 cup diced tomatoes (fresh or canned, no•salt•added)
• 1/2 cup cooked quinoa
• 2 tbsp chopped fresh basil
• 1 tsp dried oregano
• 1/4 tsp salt
• 1/4 tsp black pepper
• 1/2 cup shredded part•skim mozzarella cheese

Instructions:

1. Preheat oven to 400°F. Lightly grease a baking sheet or oven•safe dish.

2. Arrange the portobello mushroom caps, gill•side up, on the prepared baking sheet.

3. In a large skillet, cook the ground turkey over medium heat, breaking it up as It cooks, until no longer pink, about 5•7 minutes.

4. Add the chopped mushroom stems, onion, and garlic to the skillet. Cook for an additional 3•4 minutes, until the onion is translucent.

5. Stir in the diced tomatoes, cooked quinoa, basil, oregano, salt, and black pepper. Cook for 2•3 minutes to allow the flavors to blend.

6. Spoon the turkey and vegetable mixture evenly into the portobello mushroom caps.

7. Top each stuffed mushroom with a sprinkle of the shredded mozzarella cheese.

8. Bake for 15•20 minutes, or until the mushrooms are tender and the cheese is melted and bubbly. Serve the stuffed portobello mushrooms warm.

This stuffed portobello mushroom dish is an excellent choice for a diabetic•friendly, over 50 diet. The lean ground turkey provides a good source of protein, while the quinoa and mushrooms add fiber and nutrients. The simple seasoning adds flavor without the need for excessive salt or sugar. This meal is well•balanced and supports healthy blood sugar management.

83. Chicken and vegetable stir•fry with cauliflower rice

Ingredient:

Stir•Fry:
• 1 lb boneless, skinless chicken breasts, cut into 1•inch pieces
• 2 tbsp low•sodium soy sauce or tamari

Cauliflower Rice:
• 1 medium head of cauliflower, riced (about 4 cups riced cauliflower)
• 1 tbsp olive oil
• 1/4 tsp salt
• 1/4 tsp black pepper

• 1 tbsp rice vinegar
• 1 tsp sesame oil
• 1 tbsp olive oil
• 2 cups mixed vegetables (such as broccoli florets, sliced bell peppers, snow peas, and sliced mushrooms)
• 2 cloves garlic, minced
• 1 tsp grated fresh ginger
• 1/4 tsp red pepper flakes (optional)

Instructions:

1. In a small bowl, whisk together the soy sauce, rice vinegar, and sesame oil. Set aside.

2. Heat the 1 tbsp olive oil in a large skillet or wok over high heat.

3. Add the chicken pieces and stir•fry for 5•7 minutes, until the chicken is cooked through and no longer pink.

4. Add the mixed vegetables, garlic, ginger, and red pepper flakes (if using) to the skillet. Stir•fry for an additional 5•7 minutes, until the vegetables are tender•crisp.

5. Pour the soy sauce mixture into the skillet and toss everything together to coat the chicken and vegetables.

6. In a separate skillet, heat the 1 tbsp olive oil over medium heat. Add the riced cauliflower, salt, and black pepper. Sauté for 5•7 minutes, stirring occasionally, until the cauliflower rice is tender. Serve the chicken and vegetable stir•fry over the cauliflower rice.

This chicken and vegetable stir•fry with cauliflower rice is an excellent choice for a diabetic•friendly, over 50 diet. The lean chicken and variety of vegetables provide a good source of protein, fiber, and nutrients, while the cauliflower rice offers a low•carb alternative to traditional rice. The simple stir•fry sauce adds flavor without the need for excessive salt or sugar. This meal is well•balanced and supports healthy blood sugar management.

84. Baked trout with a side of roasted Brussels sprouts

Ingredient:

Trout:
• 4 (6 oz) trout fillets
• 2 tbsp olive oil
• 1 tsp lemon zest
• 2 tbsp lemon juice
• 1 tsp dried dill
• 1/4 tsp salt
• 1/4 tsp black pepper

Brussels Sprouts:
• 1 lb Brussels sprouts, trimmed and halved
• 2 tbsp olive oil
• 1 tsp garlic powder
• 1/4 tsp salt
• 1/4 tsp black pepper

Instructions:

1. Preheat oven to 400°F. Line a baking sheet with parchment paper.

2. In a small bowl, whisk together the 2 tbsp olive oil, lemon zest, lemon juice, dried dill, salt, and black pepper.

3. Place the trout fillets on the prepared baking sheet. Spoon the lemon•herb mixture over the top of the trout, making sure to evenly coat each fillet.

4. In a separate bowl, toss the Brussels sprouts with the 2 tbsp olive oil, garlic powder, salt, and black pepper.

5. Arrange the seasoned Brussels sprouts around the trout fillets on the baking sheet.

6. Bake for 15•20 minutes, or until the trout is opaque and flakes easily with a fork, and the Brussels sprouts are tender and lightly browned. Serve the baked trout immediately, with the roasted Brussels sprouts on the side.

This baked trout with roasted Brussels sprouts dish is an excellent choice for a diabetic•friendly, over 50 diet. Trout is a lean, high•protein fish that is low in carbs and calories. The Brussels sprouts provide fiber, vitamins, and minerals, while the simple seasoning adds flavor without the need for excessive salt or sugar. This meal is well•balanced and supports healthy blood sugar management.

85. Turkey and vegetable meatballs with spaghetti squash

Ingredient:

Meatballs:
- 1 lb ground turkey
- 1/2 cup finely chopped onion
- 1/2 cup finely chopped bell pepper
- 1/2 cup grated zucchini
- 2 cloves garlic, minced
- 1 egg, lightly beaten
- 1/4 cup whole wheat breadcrumbs
- 2 tbsp chopped fresh parsley
- 1 tsp dried oregano
- 1/4 tsp salt
- 1/4 tsp black pepper

Spaghetti Squash:
- 1 medium spaghetti squash, halved lengthwise and seeds removed
- 1 tbsp olive oil
- 1/4 tsp salt
- 1/4 tsp black pepper

Instructions:

1. Preheat oven to 400°F. Line a baking sheet with parchment paper.

2. In a large bowl, combine all the meatball ingredients and mix well until fully incorporated.

3. Roll the meatball mixture into 1•inch balls and place them on the prepared baking sheet.

4. Bake the meatballs for 20•25 minutes, or until cooked through and lightly browned.

5. While the meatballs are baking, place the spaghetti squash halves cut•side up on a separate baking sheet. Drizzle with the olive oil and season with salt and black pepper.

6. Bake the spaghetti squash for 40•50 minutes, or until tender when pierced with a fork.

7. Remove the spaghetti squash from the oven and use a fork to gently scrape the flesh into strands, creating "spaghetti." Serve the turkey and vegetable meatballs over the spaghetti squash.

This turkey and vegetable meatball dish with spaghetti squash is an excellent choice for a diabetic•friendly, over 50 diet. The lean turkey and vegetable•packed meatballs provide a good source of protein and fiber, while the spaghetti squash offers a low•carb alternative to traditional pasta. The simple seasoning adds flavor without the need for excessive salt or sugar. This meal is well•balanced and supports healthy blood sugar management.

86. Grilled mahi-mahi with a side of quinoa

Ingredient:

Mahi•Mahi:
• 4 (6 oz) mahi•mahi fillets
• 2 tbsp olive oil
• 1 tbsp lemon juice
• 1 tsp dried oregano
• 1/2 tsp garlic powder
• 1/4 tsp salt
• 1/4 tsp black pepper

Quinoa:
• 1 cup uncooked quinoa, rinsed
• 2 cups low•sodium vegetable or chicken broth
• 1 tbsp chopped fresh parsley

Instructions:

1. Preheat grill or grill pan to medium•high heat.

2. In a shallow dish, whisk together the olive oil, lemon juice, oregano, garlic powder, salt, and black pepper. Add the mahi•mahi fillets and gently toss to coat them evenly with the marinade.

3. In a medium saucepan, combine the quinoa and broth. Bring to a boil, then reduce heat to low, cover, and simmer for 15•20 minutes, until quinoa is tender and liquid is absorbed.

4. Grill the marinated mahi•mahi fillets for 3•4 minutes per side, or until the fish flakes easily with a fork and is opaque throughout.

5. Fluff the cooked quinoa with a fork and stir in the chopped fresh parsley.

6. Serve the grilled mahi•mahi fillets over the quinoa.

This grilled mahi•mahi with quinoa dish is an excellent choice for a diabetic•friendly, over 50 diet. Mahi•mahi is a lean, high•protein fish that is low in carbs and calories. The quinoa provides complex carbohydrates, fiber, and additional nutrients. The simple seasoning adds flavor without the need for excessive salt or sugar. This meal is well•balanced and supports healthy blood sugar management.

87. Beef and vegetable stew with turnips

Ingredient:

- 1 lb beef stew meat, cut into 1·inch cubes
- 2 tbsp olive oil
- 1 onion, diced
- 1 tsp dried thyme
- 1/2 tsp dried rosemary
- 1/4 tsp black pepper
- Salt to taste (optional)
- 2 tbsp chopped fresh parsley (for garnish)
- 3 cloves garlic, minced
- 2 cups low·sodium beef broth
- 1 (14.5 oz) can no·salt·added diced tomatoes
- 2 medium turnips, peeled and cut into 1·inch cubes
- 2 carrots, peeled and sliced
- 2 celery stalks, sliced
- 1 bay leaf

Instructions:

1. In a large pot or Dutch oven, heat the olive oil over medium·high heat.

2. Add the beef cubes and brown them on all sides, about 5·7 minutes. Transfer the browned beef to a plate and set aside.

3. Reduce the heat to medium and add the onion to the pot. Cook for 3·4 minutes, until the onion is translucent.

4. Stir in the garlic and cook for an additional minute, until fragrant.

5. Add the beef broth, diced tomatoes, turnips, carrots, celery, bay leaf, thyme, rosemary, and black pepper. Bring the mixture to a boil.

6. Reduce the heat to low, cover the pot, and simmer for 45·60 minutes, or until the beef and vegetables are tender.

7. Remove the bay leaf. Taste the stew and add salt if needed. Serve the beef and vegetable stew hot, garnished with chopped fresh parsley.

This beef and vegetable stew with turnips is an excellent choice for a diabetic·friendly, over 50 diet. The lean beef provides a good source of protein, while the turnips, carrots, and celery add fiber, vitamins, and minerals. The simple seasoning adds flavor without the need for excessive salt or sugar. This hearty and nourishing stew is well·balanced and supports healthy blood sugar management.

88. Grilled chicken with a side of quinoa salad

Ingredient:

Grilled Chicken:
- 4 (4•oz) boneless, skinless chicken breasts
- 1 tbsp olive oil
- 1 tsp garlic powder
- 1 tsp dried oregano
- Salt and pepper to taste

Quinoa Salad:
- 1 cup cooked quinoa, cooled
- 1 cup diced cucumber
- 1 cup cherry tomatoes, halved
- 1/4 cup diced red onion
- 2 tbsp chopped fresh parsley
- 2 tbsp lemon juice
- 1 tbsp olive oil
- Salt and pepper to taste

Instructions:

1. Preheat grill or grill pan to medium•high heat.

2. In a small bowl, combine the olive oil, garlic powder, oregano, salt, and pepper. Rub the mixture all over the chicken breasts.

3. Grill the chicken for 4•5 minutes per side, or until cooked through and no longer pink in the center. Transfer to a plate and let rest for 5 minutes.

4. In a large bowl, combine the cooked quinoa, cucumber, cherry tomatoes, red onion, and parsley.

5. In a small bowl, whisk together the lemon juice and olive oil. Season with salt and pepper.

6. Drizzle the lemon•olive oil dressing over the quinoa salad and toss to coat.

7. Serve the grilled chicken alongside the quinoa salad.

This recipe is diabetic•friendly as it is high in protein from the chicken, contains a complex carbohydrate in the quinoa, and features a variety of fresh vegetables. The portion sizes are also appropriate for individuals over 50. Enjoy!

89. Pan - seared tuna with a side of mixed greens

Ingredient:

• 4 (4•oz) tuna steaks
• 1 tbsp olive oil
• 1 tsp lemon pepper seasoning
• 4 cups mixed greens (such as spinach, arugula, and kale)
• 1 cup cherry tomatoes, halved
• 1/4 cup sliced cucumber
• 2 tbsp balsamic vinegar
• 1 tbsp olive oil
• Salt and pepper to taste

Instructions:

1. Pat the tuna steaks dry with paper towels and season both sides with the lemon pepper seasoning.

2. Heat 1 tbsp of olive oil in a large skillet over medium•high heat. Add the tuna steaks and cook for 2•3 minutes per side, or until lightly seared on the outside but still pink in the center. Transfer the tuna to a plate.

3. In a large bowl, combine the mixed greens, cherry tomatoes, and sliced cucumber.

4. In a small bowl, whisk together the balsamic vinegar and 1 tbsp of olive oil. Season with salt and pepper.

5. Drizzle the balsamic vinaigrette over the salad and toss to coat.

6. Serve the pan•seared tuna steaks alongside the mixed green salad.

This recipe is diabetic•friendly as it is high in protein from the tuna, low in carbs, and features a variety of nutrient•dense greens. The portion sizes are also appropriate for individuals over 50. Enjoy!

90. Vegetarian lentil loaf with a side of mashed cauliflower

Ingredient:

Lentil Loaf:
• 1 cup cooked brown lentils
• 1 cup rolled oats
• 1/2 cup finely chopped onion
• 1/2 cup finely chopped mushrooms
• 1/4 cup grated carrot
• 2 cloves garlic, minced
• 1 tsp dried thyme
• 1 tsp dried basil
• 1/4 tsp cayenne pepper (optional)
• Salt and pepper to taste

Mashed Cauliflower:
• 1 head of cauliflower, cut into florets
• 2 tbsp unsweetened almond milk
• 1 tbsp olive oil
• 1 tsp garlic powder
• Salt and pepper to taste

Instructions:

Lentil Loaf:
1. Preheat the oven to 375°F. Grease a 9x5•inch loaf pan.
2. In a large bowl, combine all the lentil loaf ingredients and mix well.
3. Transfer the mixture to the prepared loaf pan and bake for 40•45 minutes, or until the top is lightly browned.
4. Let the loaf cool for 10 minutes before slicing.

Mashed Cauliflower:
1. In a large pot, bring water to a boil. Add the cauliflower florets and cook until tender, about 10•12 minutes.
2. Drain the cauliflower and return it to the pot. Add the almond milk, olive oil, garlic powder, salt, and pepper.
3. Mash the cauliflower with a potato masher or immersion blender until smooth and creamy.

Serve the sliced lentil loaf alongside the mashed cauliflower.

This recipe is diabetic•friendly as it is high in fiber from the lentils and cauliflower, low in carbs, and provides a good source of plant•based protein. The portion sizes are also appropriate for individuals over 50. Enjoy!

91. Sliced bell peppers with hummus

Ingredient:

• 2 medium bell peppers (any color), sliced into strips
• 1/2 cup store•bought or homemade hummus

Instructions:

1. Wash the bell peppers and slice them into long, thin strips.

2. Arrange the bell pepper strips on a serving plate or platter.

3. Scoop the hummus into a small bowl and place it in the center of the plate, or serve the hummus alongside the bell pepper strips.

That's it! This is a quick and easy snack or appetizer that is perfect for a diabetic diet.

Benefits:

• Bell peppers are low in carbs and high in fiber, vitamins, and antioxidants.

• Hummus is a good source of plant•based protein, fiber, and healthy fats.

• The combination of the crunchy bell peppers and creamy hummus provides a satisfying and nutritious snack.

• The portion sizes are appropriate for individuals over 50 and can be easily adjusted to individual needs.

92. Celery sticks with almond butter

Ingredient:
• 4•5 celery stalks, cut into 3•4 inch sticks
• 2 tablespoons unsweetened almond butter

Instructions:

1. Wash the celery stalks and pat them dry with a paper towel.

2. Cut the celery stalks into 3•4 inch sticks.

3. Scoop the almond butter into a small bowl or ramekin.

4. Arrange the celery sticks around the almond butter for dipping.

That's it! This simple snack is perfect for a diabetic diet for individuals over 50.

Benefits:
• Celery is a low•carb, high•fiber vegetable that is rich in vitamins and minerals.

• Almond butter is a good source of healthy fats, proteln, and fiber, which can help regulate blood sugar levels.

• The combination of the crunchy celery and creamy almond butter provides a satisfying and nutritious snack.

• The portion sizes are appropriate for individuals over 50 and can be easily adjusted to individual needs.

This snack is easy to prepare, portable, and can be enjoyed as a healthy snack or light meal. Enjoy!

93. Mixed nuts and seeds

Ingredient:

- 1/4 cup raw almonds
- 1/4 cup raw walnuts
- 1/4 cup raw pumpkin seeds
- 1/4 cup raw sunflower seeds
- 1 tbsp chia seeds
- 1 tbsp ground flaxseeds
- 1/4 tsp ground cinnamon (optional)
- Pinch of sea salt (optional)

Instructions:

1. In a small bowl, combine the almonds, walnuts, pumpkin seeds, sunflower seeds, chia seeds, and ground flaxseeds.

2. If desired, sprinkle the mixture with ground cinnamon and a pinch of sea salt. Stir to combine.

3. Divide the mixed nuts and seeds into individual servings, such as 1/4 cup portions, and store in airtight containers.

This mixed nuts and seeds snack is perfect for a diabetic diet for individuals over 50 for the following reasons:

• Nuts and seeds are high in healthy fats, protein, fiber, and various vitamins and minerals, which can help regulate blood sugar levels and provide sustained energy.

• The combination of different nuts and seeds offers a variety of nutrients and textures.

• The portion size of 1/4 cup is appropriate for individuals over 50 and can be easily adjusted to individual needs.

• The snack is easy to prepare and can be stored for convenient, on•the•go snacking.

• The optional addition of cinnamon and a pinch of salt can enhance the flavor without adding significant amounts of sugar or sodium.

Enjoy this nutritious and satisfying mixed nuts and seeds snack as part of a balanced diabetic•friendly diet.

94. Apple slices with peanut butter

Ingredient:
• 1 medium apple, cored and sliced into thin wedges
• 2 tbsp natural peanut butter (no added sugar)

Instructions:
1. Wash and slice the apple into thin wedges, removing the core.

2. Spread about 1·2 tsp of peanut butter onto each apple slice.

Nutritional Information (per serving):
• Calories: 125
• Total Carbs: 12g
• Fiber: 3g
• Net Carbs: 9g
• Protein: 5g
• Fat: 8g

This recipe is a great snack option for individuals with diabetes as it provides a balance of complex carbs, fiber, protein and healthy fats from the apple and peanut butter. The fiber and protein help slow the absorption of the carbs, preventing blood sugar spikes. Be sure to choose a natural peanut butter without added sugars. Enjoy this simple, nutritious treat!

95. Greek yogurt with a handful of berries

Ingredient:

• 1 cup plain, unsweetened Greek yogurt
• 1/2 cup mixed berries (such as blueberries, raspberries, blackberries)

Instructions:

1. Scoop the Greek yogurt into a bowl.

2. Top the yogurt with the mixed berries.

Nutritional Information (per serving):
• Calories: 150
• Total Carbs: 12g
• Fiber: 3g
• Net Carbs: 9g
• Protein: 15g
• Fat: 5g

This snack is an excellent choice for individuals with diabetes. The Greek yogurt provides a good source of protein, which helps stabilize blood sugar levels. The berries add natural sweetness and fiber, which also helps prevent blood sugar spikes.

Greek yogurt is a great dairy option for those with diabetes as it is higher in protein and lower in carbs compared to regular yogurt. Be sure to choose an unsweetened variety to avoid added sugars.

This simple, nutrient•dense snack is a great way for individuals over 50 with diabetes to satisfy their sweet tooth in a healthy way. Enjoy!

96. Carrot sticks with guacamole

Ingredient:

- 1 medium avocado, mashed
- 2 tbsp diced tomato
- 1 tbsp diced onion
- 1 tbsp chopped cilantro (optional)
- 1 tbsp lime juice
- 1/4 tsp salt
- 1/4 tsp ground cumin
- 6•8 medium carrots, peeled and cut into sticks

Instructions:

1. In a small bowl, combine the mashed avocado, diced tomato, onion, cilantro (if using), lime juice, salt, and cumin. Mix well to make the guacamole.

2. Wash and peel the carrots, then cut them into sticks.

3. Serve the carrot sticks alongside the guacamole for dipping.

Nutritional Information (per serving, about 1/4 cup guacamole with 6•8 carrot sticks):

- Calories: 120
- Total Carbs: 12g
- Fiber: 6g
- Net Carbs: 6g
- Protein: 2g
- Fat: 8g

This snack is an excellent choice for individuals with diabetes. The carrots provide fiber and complex carbs, while the guacamole offers healthy fats, fiber, and antioxidants from the avocado, tomato, and onion. The combination of nutrients helps to regulate blood sugar levels.

Carrot sticks and guacamole make a satisfying, nutrient•dense snack that is suitable for a diabetic diet, especially for individuals over 50 who may have additional dietary considerations.

97. Cottage cheese with pineapple chunks

Ingredient:

• 1 cup low•fat or non•fat cottage cheese
• 1/2 cup fresh pineapple chunks

Instructions:

1. Scoop the cottage cheese into a bowl.

2. Top the cottage cheese with the fresh pineapple chunks.

Nutritional Information (per serving):
• Calories: 150
• Total Carbs: 12g
• Fiber: 2g
• Net Carbs: 10g
• Protein: 15g
• Fat: 3g

This snack is an excellent choice for individuals with diabetes. The cottage cheese provides a good source of protein, which helps stabilize blood sugar levels. The pineapple adds natural sweetness and fiber, which also helps prevent blood sugar spikes.

Cottage cheese is a great dairy option for those with diabetes as it is higher in protein and lower in carbs compared to other dairy products. Be sure to choose a low•fat or non•fat variety to keep the calorie and fat content in check.

Pineapple is a diabetic•friendly fruit as it contains natural sugars along with fiber, which helps slow the absorption of the carbs. The combination of cottage cheese and pineapple makes for a satisfying, nutrient•dense snack that is suitable for a diabetic diet, especially for individuals over 50 who may have additional dietary considerations.

98. Cherry tomatoes with mozzarella balls

Ingredient:
- 10•12 cherry tomatoes, halved
- 1/4 cup fresh mozzarella balls (or cubed mozzarella)
- 1 tbsp balsamic glaze (optional)
- Fresh basil leaves, chopped (optional)
- Salt and pepper to taste

Instructions:
1. Wash the cherry tomatoes and slice them in half.

2. Arrange the tomato halves on a plate and top with the mozzarella balls.

3. Drizzle the balsamic glaze over the top (if using).

4. Sprinkle with chopped fresh basil leaves (if using) and season with salt and pepper to taste.

Nutritional Information (per serving, about 6 tomato halves with 2 tbsp mozzarella):
- Calories: 90
- Total Carbs: 5g
- Fiber: 1g
- Net Carbs: 4g
- Protein: 7g
- Fat: 5g

This snack is an excellent choice for individuals with diabetes. The cherry tomatoes provide fiber, vitamins, and antioxidants, while the mozzarella cheese offers protein and healthy fats to help stabilize blood sugar levels.

The combination of the juicy tomatoes, creamy mozzarella, and optional balsamic glaze and basil creates a flavorful and satisfying snack that is suitable for a diabetic diet, especially for individuals over 50 who may have additional dietary considerations.

Remember to choose fresh, high•quality ingredients and adjust the portion sizes as needed to fit your individual dietary needs.

99. Hard - boiled eggs

Ingredient:
- Large eggs
- Water

Instructions:

1. Place the eggs in a single layer in a saucepan and cover with cold water by 1 inch.

2. Bring the water to a boil over high heat. Once the water reaches a full boil, remove the pan from the heat and cover.

3. Let the eggs sit in the hot water for 12 minutes for large eggs. Adjust the time up or down by a minute or two for smaller or larger eggs.

4. Drain the hot water and cover the eggs with cold water to stop the cooking. Let sit for 5 minutes.

5. Peel the eggs and enjoy! Store any leftover hard•boiled eggs in the refrigerator for up to 1 week.

Tips:
- Eggs are an excellent source of protein and nutrients for a diabetic diet.
- Hard•boiling the eggs is a simple way to prepare them without added fats or sugars.
- Pair the hard•boiled eggs with other diabetic•friendly foods like vegetables, whole grains, or a small portion of fruit for a balanced snack or meal.

100. Edamame

Ingredient:
• 1 lb fresh or frozen edamame in the pod
• 1•2 tsp sea salt (optional)

Instructions:

1. Bring a large pot of water to a boil over high heat.

2. Add the edamame pods to the boiling water. Cook for 5•7 minutes, until the pods are bright green and tender.

3. Drain the edamame and transfer to a serving bowl.

4. If desired, sprinkle with a small amount of sea salt.

5. Serve the edamame warm or at room temperature. Provide small bowls for discarding the empty pods.

Tips:
• Edamame is a great diabetic•friendly snack or side dish. It's high In fiber, protein, and nutrients, and low in carbs.

• The salt is optional • the edamame has a naturally savory flavor on its own.

• For a flavor twist, you can also season the cooked edamame with a small amount of soy sauce, lemon juice, or other spices.

• Pair the edamame with other lean proteins, non•starchy vegetables, and whole grains for a balanced diabetic•friendly meal.

101. Sugar - free gelatin

Ingredient:

• 1 (0.25 oz) packet of unflavored gelatin
• 2 cups unsweetened fruit juice or water
• 1•2 packets of zero•calorie sweetener (optional)

Instructions:

1. Pour the fruit juice or water into a medium saucepan. Sprinkle the gelatin over the top and let it sit for 2•3 minutes to bloom.

2. Place the saucepan over medium heat and whisk the mixture constantly until the gelatin has fully dissolved, about 2•3 minutes. Do not boil.

3. Remove the pan from the heat. If using a sweetener, add 1•2 packets now and stir to dissolve.

4. Pour the gelatin mixture into a lightly oiled 8x8 inch baking dish or individual ramekins.

5. Refrigerate for at least 4 hours, or until the gelatin is fully set.

6. Once set, cut into cubes or scoop into servings.

Tips:
• Use unsweetened fruit juices like apple, grape, or cranberry for added flavor and nutrients.

• The zero•calorie sweetener is optional if you prefer a more tart, unsweetened gelatin.

• Serve the sugar•free gelatin on its own or topped with fresh berries for a diabetic•friendly dessert.

• Store any leftover gelatin in the refrigerator for up to 1 week.

102. Almond flour muffins

Ingredient:
- 2 cups almond flour
- 1/2 cup granulated erythritol or other zero•calorie sweetener
- 1 tsp baking powder
- 1/4 tsp salt
- 3 large eggs
- 1/4 cup unsweetened almond milk
- 2 tbsp melted coconut oil or unsalted butter
- 1 tsp vanilla extract

Instructions:

1. Preheat the oven to 350°F. Grease a 12•cup muffin tin or line with paper liners.

2. In a large bowl, whisk together the almond flour, erythritol, baking powder, and salt.

3. In a separate bowl, beat the eggs. Then stir in the almond milk, melted coconut oil, and vanilla.

4. Pour the wet ingredients into the dry ingredients and mix Just until combined, being careful not to overmix.

5. Scoop the batter evenly into the prepared muffin cups, filling them about 3/4 full.

6. Bake for 18•22 minutes, until a toothpick inserted in the center comes out clean.

7. Allow the muffins to cool in the pan for 5 minutes, then transfer to a wire rack to cool completely.

Tips:
- Almond flour is a great low•carb, high•fiber alternative to regular flour for diabetic•friendly baking.

- Erythritol is a zero•calorie sweetener that won't spike blood sugar levels.

- You can add mix•ins like blueberries, chopped nuts, or sugar•free chocolate chips for extra flavor.

- Store the muffins in an airtight container in the refrigerator for up to 1 week.

103. Kale chips

Ingredient:

- 1 bunch kale, washed and dried thoroughly
- 1•2 tbsp olive oil or avocado oil
- 1/4 tsp sea salt (or to taste)
- Optional seasonings: garlic powder, onion powder, paprika, black pepper

Instructions:

1. Preheat the oven to 325°F. Line 1•2 large baking sheets with parchment paper.

2. Tear the kale leaves into bite•sized pieces, discarding any thick stems. Place the kale in a large bowl.

3. Drizzle the kale with the oil and use your hands to massage it into the leaves, making sure they are all lightly coated.

4. Sprinkle the salt and any other desired seasonings over the kale and toss to coat evenly.

5. Arrange the kale leaves in a single layer on the prepared baking sheets, making sure they are not overlapping.

6. Bake for 12•18 minutes, flipping the kale halfway through, until the leaves are crispy and lightly browned.

7. Remove the kale chips from the oven and let cool completely before serving.

Tips:
- Kale is an excellent low•carb, nutrient•dense vegetable for a diabetic diet.

- The oil helps the kale get crispy in the oven. Use just enough to lightly coat the leaves.

- Experiment with different seasonings to find your favorite flavor combinations.

- Store any leftover kale chips in an airtight container at room temperature for up to 5 days.

104. Zucchini chips

Ingredient:
• 2 medium zucchinis, sliced into 1/8•inch thick rounds
• 1•2 tbsp olive oil or avocado oil
• 1/2 tsp sea salt
• Optional seasonings: garlic powder, onion powder, paprika, black pepper

Instructions:

1. Preheat the oven to 225°F. Line 2•3 large baking sheets with parchment paper.

2. Slice the zucchinis into thin, even rounds using a mandoline slicer or sharp knife.

3. Place the zucchini slices in a large bowl and drizzle with the oil. Toss to coat the slices evenly.

4. Arrange the zucchini slices in a single layer on the prepared baking sheets, making sure they are not overlapping.

5. Sprinkle the sea salt and any other desired seasonings over the zucchini slices.

6. Bake for 1.5•2 hours, flipping the slices halfway through, until they are crispy and lightly browned.

7. Remove the zucchini chips from the oven and let cool completely before serving.

Tips:
• Zucchini is a low•carb, high•fiber vegetable that is perfect for a diabetic diet.

• Slicing the zucchini very thin is key to getting them crispy in the oven.

• Use just enough oil to lightly coat the slices • you don't want them to be greasy.

• Experiment with different seasoning blends to find your favorite flavor.

• Store any leftover zucchini chips in an airtight container at room temperature for up to 5 days.

105. Avocado chocolate mousse

Ingredient:

- 2 ripe avocados, pitted and flesh scooped out
- 1/2 cup unsweetened cocoa powder
- 1/4 cup unsweetened almond milk
- 2•3 tbsp zero•calorie sweetener (such as erythritol or stevia)
- 1 tsp vanilla extract
- 1/4 tsp sea salt

Instructions:

1. In a food processor or high•powered blender, combine the avocado flesh, cocoa powder, almond milk, sweetener, vanilla, and salt. Blend until completely smooth and creamy, scraping down the sides as needed.

2. Taste and adjust sweetener as desired, blending again to incorporate.

3. Transfer the chocolate mousse to individual serving dishes or ramekins. Cover and refrigerate for at least 2 hours, or until set.

4. Serve chilled, garnished with a sprinkle of cocoa powder, chopped nuts, or fresh berries if desired.

Tips:
- Avocados provide healthy fats, fiber, and creaminess to this diabetic•friendly dessert.

- The unsweetened cocoa powder and zero•calorie sweetener keep the carbs and sugar low.

- Almond milk adds richness without dairy.

- This mousse can be made up to 3 days in advance and stored in the refrigerator.

- For a thicker consistency, use less almond milk. For a thinner texture, add a bit more.

106. Fresh fruit salad with mint

Ingredient:
- 1 cup diced watermelon
- 1 cup diced pineapple
- 1 cup diced strawberries
- 1 cup diced mango
- 1/4 cup fresh mint leaves, chopped
- 1 tbsp fresh lime juice
- 1 tsp zero•calorie sweetener (optional)

Instructions:

1. In a large bowl, combine the diced watermelon, pineapple, strawberries, and mango.

2. Add the chopped mint leaves and drizzle the lime juice over the fruit.

3. If desired, sprinkle the zero•calorie sweetener over the fruit salad and gently toss to combine.

4. Cover and refrigerate for at least 30 minutes to allow the flavors to meld.

5. Serve the fresh fruit salad chilled.

Tips:
• This fruit salad is packed with vitamins, minerals, and antioxidants that are great for a diabetic diet.

• The zero•calorie sweetener is optional if you prefer a more tart, unsweetened fruit salad.

• You can use any combination of fresh, in•season fruits that you enjoy.

• The mint adds a refreshing, aromatic element to the salad.

• Serve the fruit salad on its own or with a dollop of plain Greek yogurt for added protein.

• Store any leftover salad in the refrigerator for up to 3 days.

107. Coconut flour cookies

Ingredient:

- 1/2 cup coconut flour
- 1/4 cup granulated erythritol or other zero•calorie sweetener
- 1/4 tsp baking soda
- 1/4 tsp sea salt
- 3 large eggs
- 1/4 cup melted coconut oil or unsalted butter
- 1 tsp vanilla extract

Instructions:

1. Preheat the oven to 350°F. Line a baking sheet with parchment paper.

2. In a medium bowl, whisk together the coconut flour, erythritol, baking soda, and salt.

3. In a separate bowl, beat the eggs. Then stir in the melted coconut oil and vanilla.

4. Pour the wet ingredients into the dry ingredients and mix until a thick dough forms.

5. Scoop the dough by the tablespoonful onto the prepared baking sheet, spacing them about 2 inches apart.

6. Bake for 12•15 minutes, until the cookies are lightly golden around the edges.

7. Allow the cookies to cool on the baking sheet for 5 minutes before transferring to a wire rack to cool completely.

Tips:
- Coconut flour is a great low•carb, high•fiber alternative to regular flour for diabetic•friendly baking.

- Erythritol is a zero•calorie sweetener that won't spike blood sugar levels.

- You can add mix•ins like chopped nuts, unsweetened shredded coconut, or sugar•free chocolate chips.

- Store the cookies in an airtight container at room temperature for up to 1 week.

108. Baked apple with cinnamon

Ingredient:
• 4 medium apples, cored (such as Gala, Fuji, or Honeycrisp)
• 1/4 cup water
• 2 tbsp unsweetened applesauce
• 1 tsp ground cinnamon
• 1/4 tsp ground nutmeg (optional)
• 1 tbsp chopped walnuts or pecans (optional)
• 1 tbsp zero•calorie sweetener (such as erythritol or stevia), optional

Instructions:

1. Preheat the oven to 375°F. Lightly grease a baking dish or line with parchment paper.

2. Core the apples, leaving the bottom intact so they can stand upright. Place the apples in the prepared baking dish.

3. In a small bowl, mix together the water, applesauce, cinnamon, and nutmeg (if using). Pour this mixture over and around the apples.

4. If using the sweetener, sprinkle it evenly over the tops of the apples.

5. Bake for 30•40 minutes, until the apples are tender when pierced with a fork.

6. Remove the apples from the oven and let cool for 5 minutes.

7. Serve the baked apples warm, drizzled with the cinnamon•spiced sauce. Top with chopped nuts if desired.

Tips:
• Apples are a great source of fiber, vitamins, and antioxidants for a diabetic diet.

• The applesauce and cinnamon add sweetness without added sugar.

• The optional sweetener can be used if you prefer a sweeter dessert.

• Pair the baked apples with a dollop of unsweetened Greek yogurt for added protein.

• Store any leftover baked apples in the refrigerator for up to 3 days.

109. Dark chocolate squares (in moderation)

Ingredient:

- 4 oz high•quality dark chocolate (at least 70% cacao), chopped
- 1 tbsp coconut oil
- 1/4 tsp sea salt (optional)

Instructions:

1. Line a small baking sheet or 8x8 inch baking pan with parchment paper.

2. In a double boiler or heatproof bowl set over a saucepan of simmering water, melt the chopped dark chocolate and coconut oil, stirring frequently until smooth.

3. Remove the melted chocolate mixture from the heat. Stir in the sea salt, if using.

4. Pour the chocolate into the prepared pan, spreading it evenly.

5. Refrigerate for at least 2 hours, or until the chocolate is completely set.

6. Once set, break or cut the chocolate into 16 equal squares.

7. Store the dark chocolate squares in an airtight container in the refrigerator for up to 2 weeks.

Tips:
- Dark chocolate with a high cacao percentage is lower in sugar and carbs compared to milk chocolate.

- Coconut oil helps the chocolate set up nicely without any added sugar.

- Enjoy 1•2 squares of the dark chocolate as an occasional treat, as part of a balanced diabetic diet.

- The sea salt is optional, but it can help balance the bitterness of the dark chocolate.

- You can customize the squares by adding a sprinkle of chopped nuts, unsweetened shredded coconut, or a light dusting of cocoa powder.

110. Chia seed pudding with almond milk

Ingredient:
- 1/4 cup chia seeds
- 1 cup unsweetened almond milk
- 1•2 tbsp zero•calorie sweetener (such as erythritol or stevia)
- 1 tsp vanilla extract
- 1/4 tsp ground cinnamon (optional)
- Fresh berries or sliced almonds for topping (optional)

Instructions:

1. In a medium bowl, whisk together the chia seeds, almond milk, sweetener, vanilla, and cinnamon (if using) until well combined.

2. Cover the bowl and refrigerate for at least 4 hours, or overnight, stirring occasionally, until the mixture has thickened to a pudding•like consistency.

3. Divide the chia seed pudding into individual serving bowls or jars.

4. Top with fresh berries, sliced almonds, or any other desired toppings.

5. Serve chilled.

Tips:
- Chia seeds are an excellent source of fiber, protein, and healthy omega•3 fatty acids, making them a great choice for a diabetic diet.

- Unsweetened almond milk is low in carbs and calories compared to regular dairy milk.

- Start with 1 tbsp of sweetener and add more to taste, depending on your preference.

- The cinnamon adds a warm, comforting flavor, but is optional.

- This pudding can be made in advance and stored in the refrigerator for up to 5 days.

- For a thicker consistency, use 1/3 cup chia seeds instead of 1/4 cup.

111. Roasted chickpeas

Ingredient:

- 1 (15 oz) can chickpeas (garbanzo beans), drained and rinsed
- 1 tbsp olive oil
- 1/2 tsp ground cumin
- 1/2 tsp paprika
- 1/4 tsp garlic powder
- 1/4 tsp sea salt

Instructions:

1. Preheat the oven to 400°F. Line a baking sheet with parchment paper.

2. Pat the drained and rinsed chickpeas very dry with paper towels or a clean kitchen towel.

3. In a medium bowl, toss the chickpeas with the olive oil, cumin, paprika, garlic powder, and salt until evenly coated.

4. Spread the chickpeas in a single layer on the prepared baking sheet.

5. Roast for 20•25 minutes, shaking the pan halfway through, until the chickpeas are crispy and golden brown.

6. Remove the roasted chickpeas from the oven and let cool for 5 minutes before serving.

Tips:
- Chickpeas are a great source of fiber, protein, and complex carbs for a diabetic diet.

- The spices add flavor without any added sugar.

- Roasting the chickpeas makes them crispy and satisfying as a snack or topping.

- You can experiment with different seasoning blends, such as chili powder, cayenne, or lemon pepper.

- Store any leftover roasted chickpeas in an airtight container at room temperature for up to 1 week.

112. Cucumber slices with tzatziki

Ingredient:

Tzatziki Dip:
• 1 cup plain Greek yogurt (full•fat or low•fat)
• 1 medium cucumber, peeled, seeded, and grated
• 1 garlic clove, minced
• 1 tbsp fresh lemon juice
• 1 tbsp chopped fresh dill
• 1/4 tsp salt

Cucumber Slices:
• 2 medium cucumbers, sliced into 1/4•inch thick rounds

Instructions:
1. Make the tzatziki dip: In a medium bowl, combine the Greek yogurt, grated cucumber, garlic, lemon juice, dill, and salt. Stir until well mixed. Cover and refrigerate for at least 30 minutes to allow the flavors to blend.

2. Arrange the cucumber slices on a serving platter or plate.

3. Serve the chilled tzatziki dip alongside the cucumber slices for dipping.

Tips:
• Cucumbers are a low•calorie, low•carb vegetable that is hydrating and rich in vitamins and minerals.

• Greek yogurt provides protein and probiotics, which are important for gut health in older adults.

• The tzatziki dip is creamy and flavorful without any added sugars or unhealthy fats.

• This snack is a great option for individuals over 50 with diabetes, as it is low in carbs and high in nutrients.

• You can also serve the tzatziki with other raw veggies like bell peppers, carrots, or cherry tomatoes.

• Store any leftover tzatziki in the refrigerator for up to 5 days.

113. Homemade trail mix with nuts and dried fruit

Ingredient:

- 1/2 cup raw almonds
- 1/2 cup raw walnuts
- 1/4 cup raw pecans
- 1/4 cup unsweetened shredded coconut
- 2 tbsp unsweetened dried cranberries
- 2 tbsp unsweetened dried blueberries
- 1 tbsp unsweetened cacao nibs (optional)
- 1/4 tsp ground cinnamon

Instructions:

1. In a large bowl, combine the almonds, walnuts, pecans, shredded coconut, dried cranberries, dried blueberries, and cacao nibs (if using).

2. Sprinkle the cinnamon over the top and stir gently to mix everything together.

3. Transfer the trail mix to an airtight container or resealable bag.

4. Store the trail mix at room temperature for up to 2 weeks.

Tips:
- Nuts are a great source of healthy fats, protein, and fiber for a diabetic diet.

- Dried berries provide natural sweetness without added sugars.

- The cacao nibs add a rich chocolate flavor and antioxidants.

- Cinnamon may help regulate blood sugar levels.

- Portion out the trail mix into 1/4 cup servings to control portion sizes.

- You can customize the mix by using different nuts and dried fruits you enjoy.

- Avoid trail mixes with added sugars, oils, or candies.

114. Berry smoothie with protein powder

Ingredient:

- 1 cup unsweetened almond milk
- 1/2 cup frozen mixed berries (such as blueberries, raspberries, and blackberries)
- 1 scoop vanilla or unflavored protein powder (about 20•25 grams)
- 1 tbsp ground flaxseed
- 1 tsp honey or zero•calorie sweetener (optional)
- 1/2 cup ice cubes

Instructions:

1. Add all the ingredients to a high•powered blender. Blend on high speed until smooth and creamy, about 1 minute.

2. Taste and adjust sweetener if desired. Blend again briefly to incorporate.

3. Pour the berry smoothie into a glass and serve immediately.

Tips:
- Berries are an excellent source of antioxidants, fiber, and low•glycemic carbs for a diabetic diet.

- Protein powder helps provide sustained energy and supports muscle health.

- Flaxseed adds healthy omega•3 fatty acids and extra fiber.

- Use an unsweetened almond milk to keep the carbs low. Dairy milk can also be used.

- The honey or zero•calorie sweetener is optional if you prefer a less sweet smoothie.

- For a thicker consistency, use more frozen berries or less almond milk.

- You can also add a handful of spinach or kale for extra nutrients.

115. Sugar•free popsicles

Ingredient:

- 2 cups unsweetened fruit juice (such as apple, grape, or berry)
- 1/4 cup unsweetened almond milk or coconut milk
- 1•2 tbsp zero•calorie sweetener (such as erythritol or stevia)
- 1 tsp lemon or lime juice (optional)

Instructions:

1. In a medium bowl, whisk together the fruit juice, almond/coconut milk, and zero•calorie sweetener until the sweetener is fully dissolved.

2. Stir in the lemon or lime juice, if using, to add a touch of tartness.

3. Carefully pour the mixture into popsicle molds, leaving a small amount of headspace at the top.

4. Insert popsicle sticks and freeze for at least 4 hours, or until completely solid.

5. To remove the popsicles, run the molds under warm water for 30 seconds to 1 minute, then gently pull the popsicles out.

Tips:
- Use unsweetened fruit juices to provide natural sweetness and flavor without added sugars.

- The almond or coconut milk adds creaminess and helps create a smooth, icy texture.

- Start with 1 tbsp of sweetener and add more to taste, depending on the sweetness of the fruit juice.

- You can experiment with different juice and milk combinations, such as strawberry•banana or pineapple•coconut.

- For extra nutrition, you can blend in a small amount of pureed fruit or vegetables.

- Store the popsicles in an airtight container in the freezer for up to 2 months.

116. Almond flour crackers with cheese

Ingredient:
• 1 1/2 cups almond flour
• 1/2 cup shredded cheddar or parmesan cheese
• 1 tbsp ground flaxseed
• 1/2 tsp garlic powder
• 1/4 tsp onion powder
• 1/4 tsp salt
• 2 tbsp unsalted butter, melted
• 1•2 tbsp water (as needed)

Instructions:

1. Preheat the oven to 350°F. Line a baking sheet with parchment paper.

2. In a medium bowl, whisk together the almond flour, shredded cheese, flaxseed, garlic powder, onion powder, and salt.

3. Pour in the melted butter and stir until the mixture starts to come together. Add 1•2 tbsp of water as needed to form a dough.

4. Roll the dough out between two sheets of parchment paper to about 1/8•inch thickness.

5. Use a sharp knife or cookie cutter to cut the dough into cracker shapes. Transfer the crackers to the prepared baking sheet, spacing them apart.

6. Bake for 12•15 minutes, flipping the crackers halfway through, until golden brown and crispy.

7. Allow the crackers to cool completely on the baking sheet before serving.

Tips:
• Almond flour is a low•carb, high•fiber alternative to regular flour for diabetic•friendly baking.
• The cheese adds flavor and a crispy texture to the crackers.
• Flaxseed provides extra fiber and healthy omega•3 fatty acids.
• Serve the crackers with slices of cheese, olives, or other low•carb toppings.
• Store any leftover crackers in an airtight container at room temeprature for up to 1 week.

117. Cauliflower popcorn

Ingredient:

- 1 head of cauliflower, cut into small florets
- 2 tbsp olive oil or avocado oil
- 1/2 tsp garlic powder
- 1/2 tsp onion powder
- 1/4 tsp smoked paprika
- 1/4 tsp salt

Instructions:

1. Preheat the oven to 400°F. Line a large baking sheet with parchment paper.

2. In a large bowl, toss the cauliflower florets with the oil, garlic powder, onion powder, smoked paprika, and salt until evenly coated.

3. Spread the seasoned cauliflower in a single layer on the prepared baking sheet.

4. Roast for 20•25 minutes, stirring halfway, until the cauliflower is tender and lightly browned.

5. Remove the cauliflower "popcorn" from the oven and let cool for 5 minutes before serving.

Tips:
- Cauliflower is a low•carb, high•fiber vegetable that makes a great alternative to traditional popcorn.

- The spices add flavor without any added sugars.

- You can experiment with different seasoning blends, such as chili powder, cumin, or lemon pepper.

- For a crispier texture, spread the cauliflower in an even layer and avoid overcrowding the baking sheet.

- Enjoy the cauliflower popcorn on its own as a snack or pair it with dips like tzatziki or hummus.

- Store any leftover cauliflower popcorn in an airtight container at room temperature for up to 3 days.

Congratulations on completing ***The Complete Diabetic Diet After 50."*** By embracing the knowledge, recipes, and meal plans provided in this book, you have taken a significant step towards better managing your prediabetes or type 2 diabetes. More importantly, you have committed to a lifestyle that prioritizes your health and well-being.

Managing diabetes is a lifelong journey, but it doesn't have to be a daunting one. This book has armed you with a wealth of delicious, low-sugar, and low-carb recipes that prove healthy eating can be both enjoyable and satisfying. You've learned how to make informed dietary choices, understand the impact of carbohydrates and sugars, and implement practical strategies for maintaining stable blood sugar levels.

The 60-day meal plan has guided you through structured, balanced eating, showing you that consistency is key to effective diabetes management. It has provided a blueprint for planning your meals in a way that supports your health goals while fitting seamlessly into your lifestyle. As you move beyond these initial 60 days, you can continue to adapt and personalize your meal plans using the principles and recipes you've mastered.

Remember, the journey to better health is ongoing, and it's perfectly normal to encounter challenges along the way. Stay patient and kind to yourself as you continue to adapt to your new dietary habits. Reach out to healthcare professionals when you need support, and connect with others who share similar experiences. Community and support networks can be invaluable in maintaining motivation and achieving long-term success.

Your journey with ***The Complete Diabetic Diet After 50"*** doesn't end here. Use this book as a continuous resource, revisiting favorite recipes, trying new ones, and refreshing your meal plans as needed. Let it inspire you to explore new foods, experiment in the kitchen, and discover the joys of healthy eating.

In closing, managing prediabetes and type 2 diabetes is about more than just diet; it's about embracing a holistic approach to health that includes regular physical activity, mental well-being, and consistent medical care. By integrating these elements into your daily life, you are well on your way to achieving a healthier, happier you.

Thank you for allowing this book to be part of your journey. May it continue to guide and inspire you as you live your healthiest life after 50. Here's to your ongoing success and well-being!
